RJ NORTHINGTON

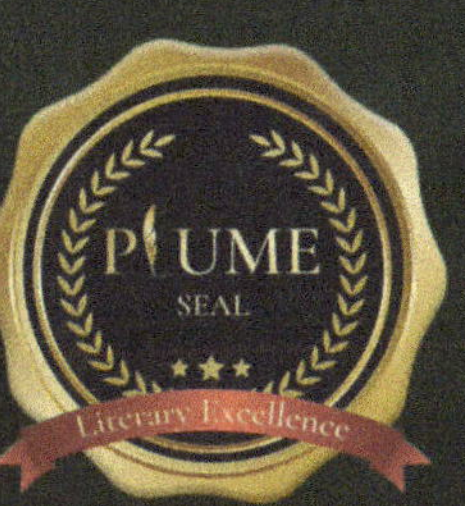

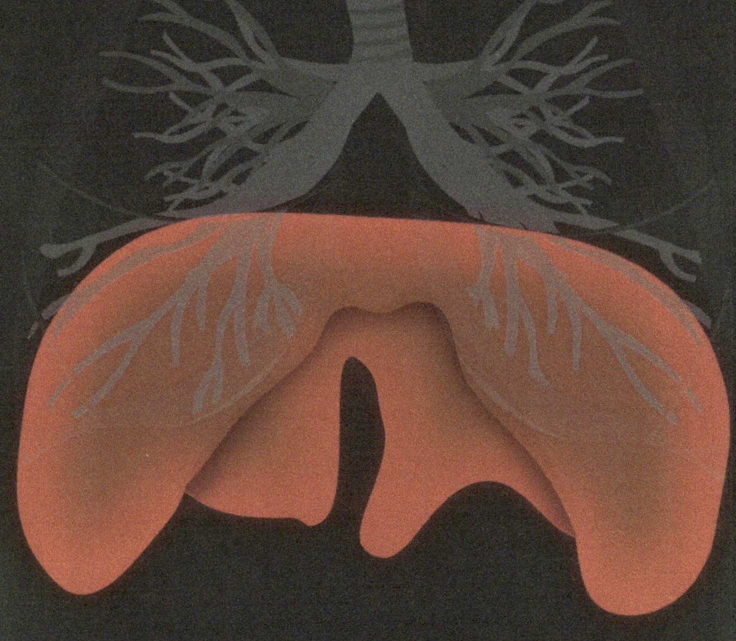

The Diaphragm

The MUSCLE SOURCE of LIFE

SECOND EDITION

ISBN 978-1-961254-63-3 (softcover)
ISBN 978-1-961254-65-7 (hardcover)
ISBN 978-1-961254-64-0 (ebook)

Printed in the United States of America.

The Diaphragm

The MUSCLE SOURCE *of* LIFE

SECOND EDITION

RJ NORTHINGTON

Table of Contents

Thank you to all that supported, encouraged, and inspired me, as well as recognized my potential.

Acknowledgement

I dedicate this book to my parents as well as myself. I take a lot of pride, and I am proud of myself in the creation of this book, as it took a lot of research, hard work, and dedication to complete. It pleases me that because of my passion and my understanding of the role of the diaphragm in bodily functions. I managed to create a piece of work that I can call my own that my parents can also be proud of. It is a piece of work that really matters and is meaningful in society, which also includes my friends and family. For many years, I wanted to be able to use the knowledge I have acquired over the years and give back. I feel so fortunate that I am now able to in educating on the diaphragm's intimate relationship with life and its influence on life altogether.

I give great thanks to my parents in their support of me in the further development and completion of this book, as it was my mom's encouraging words telling me she thinks that I should finish my writing/book and publish it in addition to my dad being impressed by what I had written that encouraged me to finish. The combination of my parents' support is what I needed to finish this book, as it was a project that was unintended and just came to be. I had to take on this project alone, as my ideas appeared to be unique and different from most people around me. A concern that I had was that I was writing ideas that felt were extent that goes beyond this version of the book. My parents' encouraging words and responses basically sealed the deal for me to get this book out there. I hope for it to be useful and beneficial for society. I am so glad I could make this book a reality. I also want to thank my parents again for always being there for me, as I know I do not thank them enough.

Qi Gong / Chi Kung Breathing
The Practice of Breath Work

It is not a waste of time if you are breathing deeply.
Abundant breath, abundant life.

Introduction

The breath is everything. The breath is life. There is no life without the breath. The breath we often associate with the air we breathe. The breath contains the very vital substance(s) needed to fuel and preserve life such as oxygen gas (oxygen, O2) and qi/chi (pronounced chee). Oxygen is the substance needed in the body to generate life-sustaining energy and qi/chi is understood as our vital energy or life force. Breathing is the act of taking breath into the body, then expelling breath out of the body, continuously, through the lungs. The taking in of breath is necessary for us to access the life sustaining substance(s) in breath in order to generate and maintain energy production for the preservation of life. The expelling of breath is necessary for the removal of waste(s) such as carbon dioxide gas (carbon dioxide, CO2) from the body. The accumulation of wastes known as metabolic wastes (wastes as a result of chemical reactions in cellular respirations) is a consequence of this energy production and needs to be removed from the body.

The act/art of breathing is very crucial in sustaining a continuous flow of breath entering and exiting our bodies in order to sustain life. This act of breathing is made possible by the function pf the thoracic diaphragm, which I will just refer to as the diaphragm. Breath only enters our body due to the contraction of the diaphragm. The breath is only expelled from our body due to the relaxation of the diaphragm. This means that the diaphragm is very vital for our access to breath and facilitation of breathing, Since the breath and breathing are very vital to life, this then means that the diaphragm is also very vital to life, as there is no breath or breathing without the function and work of the diaphragm. Therefore, the diaphragm equals life. The diaphragm is a muscle, and just like all muscles, it has a simple job/function, which is to contract and relax. The effect that a particular muscular contraction has on the body identifies its significance or purpose for the body. Yet the effects on the body from the contraction/relaxation cycle of the diaphragm function allows for the very existence of life.

The Control of the Breath

The breath or breathing is controlled by the diaphragm, and because it is a muscle, the diaphragm is only able to contract and /or relax. So in general, the contraction of the diaphragm facilitates the process of inhalation. Inhalation is known as the process of drawing in or pulling in breath (air, O_2, chi/qi, etc). The relaxation of the diaphragm facilitates the process of exhalation. Exhalation is known as the process of expelling or pushing out breath (air, O_2, chi/qi, etc). It is the inhalation process that provides the vital substance for life. It is the exhalation process that removes metabolic wastes, generated from the use of the vital substance. One inhalation paired with an exhalation is considered one breathing cycle.

The Identity and Control of the Diaphragm

More specifically, as a muscle, the diaphragm is a skeletal muscle, and skeletal muscle function under voluntary control. This means that the diaphragm should be under voluntary control. However, the uniqueness of this skeletal muscle is that even though it can be controlled by the somatic (voluntary) nervous system, it is predominately controlled by the autonomic (involuntary) nervous system. This combination of control and influence indicates the importance of the function that the diaphragm has in the body, as the diaphragm must continue to function even when we are not conscious.

The diaphragm therefore responds to these two systems of influence on its function. The diaphragm is innervated by the phrenic and intercostal nerves, nerves that are a part of the autonomic nervous system. The autonomic nervous system controls the unconscious, involuntary breathing or unconscious, involuntary contraction and relaxation of the diaphragm, and the somatic nervous system controls the conscious, voluntary breathing or conscious, voluntary contraction and relaxation of the diaphragm.

Autonomic (unconscious, involuntary) breathing operates to keep you alive so that you may exist and function. The autonomic breathing control is what keeps the rhythmic breathing occurring continuously, even while sleeping or unconscious, yet it can be influenced by the somatic (voluntary, conscious) breathing/control.

The control of the somatic nervous system in allowing somatic (conscious, voluntary) breathing possible is necessary, however, in protecting and preserving the respiratory system at times when the holding of the breath is necessary, by keeping the diaphragm in stasis. This action prevents water from entering the lungs or nose, as well as prevent gaseous irritants from getting into the nose, mouth, or lungs.

Although the act of stopping the breath is necessary at times, the time allowed is limited to about three minutes. Stopping the breath means stopping the flow of oxygen entering the body, and after about three minutes, the autonomic nervous system will override the somatic nervous system and commence breathing. This demonstrates just how important it is to keep a continuous flow of the breath entering and leaving the body. The body must breathe.

The Option of the Conscious, Voluntary Control of the Diaphragm

In addition, not only is the somatic (conscious, voluntary) breathing capable of protecting the respiratory system, the somatic breathing also operates with the potential and option to fully engage the diaphragm's contraction and relaxation with each breath taken, and upon inhalation will bring in more "breath" and upon exhalation will release more metabolic wastes. This increase in breath brings in more air, oxygen, and qi/chi into the body than what a normal autonomic involuntary diaphragmatic contractional breath would bring in. This increase in breath increases strength, power, longevity, youth, and energy production or sustain function for a longer period. This would facilitate normal bodily functions at more efficient levels. The full engagement/contraction of the diaphragm can be considered the act of taking a deep breath.

For an analogy, I would like to associate the deepness or fullness of an inhalation of breath with the degree of engagement in contraction of the diaphragm. You can readily notice that you can take a deeper inhalation when you do it unconsciously or involuntarily. This deeper inhalation is accomplished by a stronger, lengthier, more complete contraction of the diaphragm, voluntarily. This voluntary diaphragmatic contraction exceeds the contractional effort of the involuntary diaphragmatic contraction.

There must be a reason for having this option of the voluntary, conscious contraction of the diaphragm that allows us to take a voluntary, conscious breath that can exceed the amount of breath achieved by the normal involuntary, unconscious contraction of the diaphragm that occurs during involuntary unconscious breathing. It could be an option that takes us down a different path of life, a path with a limitless abundance of oxygen and chi.

We already know what happens when we allow our lives to be guided by mostly involuntary, autonomic breathing. With conscious/voluntary engagement of the diaphragm, you begin to practice the art of a "conscious" breather. It does take effort to be a conscious breather, however. And what I mean by a conscious breather is a person who contracts the diaphragm beyond their normal involuntary diaphragmatic contractional point, preferably toward a complete or maximum contraction of the diaphragm, continuously during every breathing cycle. This person then continues toward making this breathing practice a way of life.

The voluntary, conscious, full engagement of the diaphragmatic contraction puts you in the now. It is also an active process. This means it takes energy, effort, and the will. It requires consistency and a certain level of commitment to do so. It can only be performed or achieved If you want to do it. It cannot be done for you. No one else can truly breathe for you. Your breath is your life, and if you control your breath, then you control your life. Therefore, if you control your diaphragm, then you control your breath. Therefore, if you control your diaphragm then you control your life. And you have the ability to control your diaphragm. So then taking control over your diaphragm is taking control over your life. And taking control over your life includes taking control over your emotions, health, mind, body, and possibly your surroundings.

Question: Why if oxygen is something so precious that the body needs, normal contraction of the diaphragm does not exercise the ability to maximize the intake of it?

The Dependability and Resilience of the Diaphragm

The diaphragm is not a weight-bearing muscle, neither is the heart, so in consequence, they both have quick recovery periods and function continuously throughout life from birth. In other words, from birth, the diaphragm functions continuously just like the heart does. If the diaphragm ever did cease to function, we would not be able to breathe or take in breath; therefore, life as we know it would end. From this direct relationship, it makes sense to say that the more breath we take in, the greater impact on our life it should have (no breath equals no life, breath equals life, more breath equals more life, no diaphragm equals no life, diaphragm equals life, more diaphragm equals more life.)

Now the diaphragm is a skeletal muscle, and all skeletal muscles can be strengthened and developed. And due to necessity of its function, as the diaphragm is needed in any exercise you perform or during any human activity (whether it be sitting; standing; sleeping; running; walking; biking; performing arm presses, squats, and planks; etc.), the diaphragm is constantly working. Therefore. It seems very beneficial to consider the diaphragm as the main skeletal muscle to strengthen. Some benefits of strengthening the diaphragm would include the increase of total body strength, power, longevity, youth, and emotional stability for the human body, as those elements require the contents of the breath in order to manifest. Fortunately, the diaphragm has the fastest recovery time compared to other skeletal muscles allowing results to occur rather quickly.

The most notable time of "isolated" diaphragmatic activity is in doing static training. During static training, the other skeletal muscles are in stasis and you can really feel how hard the diaphragm begins to work, supplying oxygen, removing wastes, and assisting in the circulation of blood and fluids, as the diaphragm must continue to contract and relax to replace oxygen that is used up and remove wastes that build up. During dynamic training, other skeletal muscles engage long with the diaphragm and promote efficient circulation of blood and lymph, but during rest periods, those muscles are no longer engaged even if temporary unlike the diaphragm. Even after the diaphragm works hard during vigorous activity, it is still depended upon to keep working to assist in the recovery of the other muscles from fatigue as well as itself. Also, these other skeletal muscles, when active, only use up available oxygen and energy in the form of ATP (adenosine triphosphate, our energy currency), creating wastes. In support of these muscles in their active states and during their recovery periods and assist in the removal of their waste products.

The Contribution of the Diaphragm

The diaphragm's contraction cycle, whether voluntary or involuntary, is an active process. This means that on a cellular level, the contraction of the diaphragm muscle fibers require energy to contract, so they do utilize oxygen and ATP as well. However, during that process, it also facilitates the process of drawing more oxygen into the body through its effect on the lungs and thoracic cavity upon inhalation. This inhaled oxygen will then be used by the diaphragm as well as the rest of the body, including all cells. Not only will this contraction of the diaphragm provide oxygen for the whole body, but this same contraction will also increase pressure or compression on the inferior vena cava (largest vein in the body) and thoracic duct (largest lymph vessel in the body), which will result in the increase in circulation of the venous blood that returns directly into the right atrium of the heart. This contraction will also facilitate the increase in the movement of lymph fluid, the fluid that is used in the transportation system of the immune system to flow through the lymph nodes, and help its return to the circulatory system.

The diaphragm's relaxation cycle does not require energy. It relies on the natural recoiling of the elastic nature of the lungs as the diaphragm relaxes during exhalation. It will facilitate the removal of the metabolic wastes generated by the diaphragm and the rest of the cells of the body. The relaxation cycle of the diaphragm will also facilitate the increase in the circulation of the return of venous blood near the heart as well as facilitate the increase of the movement of lymph fluid by removing compression off the vessels creating space in the vessel for blood and fluid flow.

When you fall asleep, deeper breathing and slower breathing occurs in a relative sense, and the recovery of the body is phenomenal. It also does help that the muscles of the body are in a more relaxed state, not consuming much energy during sleep. Therefore, energy production exceeds energy usage during sleep. The deeper breathing that occurs can only be achieved by more engagement of the diaphragm. Be aware that when you are asleep, the intelligence of the body involuntarily increases the engagement of the contraction of the diaphragm for recovery.

This deeper act of breathing brings in more chi and oxygen to the body for increased energy production and in consequence, increases relaxation, raises strength, reduces recovery time, promotes healing, reduces stress, and may even support dreaming. It also increases the spirit, bringing you closer to the Creator, as we are considered energy or spiritual beings. If you view breath as the spirit, then the way to increase the spirit is through the breath. So to maximize the spirit would be to maximize the breath, and to maximize the breath would be to maximize diaphragmatic function.

Now if deeper breathing while asleep can increase energy, relaxation, and spirit and reduce stress, then maybe we can reap similar benefits if we mimic the same behavior of the diaphragm while awake. This would require the voluntary effort. Is breath spirit? Hmm.

The Support from the Diaphragm

The human body has its own intelligence, and when you exercise or do any rigorous physical activity, it always stimulates more involuntary activation and engagement of the diaphragm. This simulation, for more activation of the diaphragm, autonomously increase the involuntary action of the diaphragm for stronger, lengthier, almost forceful contractions and relaxations of the diaphragm at times. You will also notice that the frequency of the contraction and relaxation cycle also increase in addition to their length. It is understood that during vigorous physical activity or exercise, lots of energy is being expended and the changes in the respiratory system occur in order to adapt and keep up with the increased demand for more energy. This increase in energy production is necessary in order to provide the body with sustained strength, power, and endurance or even for more strength, power and endurance. It is oxygen that is needed to maximize energy production, and an increase in oxygen supply is necessary to provide for an increase in energy production. So when the body has a need for increased oxygen and qi/chi intake to provide for more strength, power, endurance, and energy during vigorous physical activity, there is a large dependency on the function of the diaphragm. This is evident by the increased involuntary engagement of diaphragmatic contraction in order to achieve the goal of increased oxygen intake. This sets up another equation: the diaphragm equals energy, or the diaphragm equals oxygen, or the diaphragm equals qi.

Intake of oxygen is needed to sustain body or whole body function. When an increase in energy is needed, an increase in oxygen input is needed, which would require an increase in oxygen availability and would not recommend but require more activity from the diaphragm. The body will do whatever it needs I order to maintain homeostasis with energy demands such as involve the increase in involuntary engagement of the diaphragm. It may stimulate the cramping of the other active skeletal muscles. This prevents the muscles from using up too much energy and generating too much waste or lactic acid during exercise. It may also redirect energy availability to where the body deems most vital. The muscle cramping and redirecting of energy occur when the body is unable to keep up with the energy demands meaning that the input of oxygen is not sufficient. Even regular lactic build up indicates that the oxygen input is not sufficient.

The option of the voluntary full engagement of our diaphragm at will means that we can increase our oxygen intake without the need for rigorous physical activity or the need for increased involuntary contraction of the diaphragm. The voluntary breath or voluntary contraction of the diaphragm. This voluntary breath may prevent the body from ever being in predicament to facilitate muscular cramping or energy rationing by always providing the body with an abundance of oxygen and therefore, energy.

We do not perform Vigorous activities all day, but we must breathe all day. We have the option or fully engaging our diaphragm voluntarily whenever we want tom and so we should. Oxygen nurtures the cells, and the chi protects the cells from destruction. Just like other skeletal muscles that can be developed and strengthened from physical training. The strengthening of the diaphragm can be accomplished by first becoming aware of your diaphragm and breathing pattern. When you are ready you would stimulate a near maximum or maximum muscular contraction of the diaphragm. This is also a similar training tactic you would use with any other skeletal muscles such as arms, legs, abs, etc, for strengthening purposes. This would require the diaphragmatic contractions to occur voluntarily. The voluntary training of the diaphragm is a simple yet difficult practice as it takes more mental focus than physical input. Are you fully engaging your diaphragm now as you are reading this?

Training and Strengthening of the Diaphragm

You do not have to do any vigorous running or any vigorous physical activity in order to strengthen the diaphragm, but you can. Vigorous physical activity and the voluntary control of the diaphragm both influences the diaphragm to do the same thing, which is the only thing the diaphragm can do and that is to contract and relax. Although vigorous physical activity does contribute to the increase of the involuntary contraction/engagement of the diaphragm, it is very beneficial to fully engage the diaphragm voluntarily for strengthening.

In involuntary engagement of the diaphragm from vigorous physical activity, you are not in control of your diaphragm. Contraction and relaxation cycles are rapid, which promotes sympathetic nerve activity. You also do not know if the contractions of the diaphragm are complete since they are rapid, making it hard to gauge your diaphragm's condition, but if you are in control the function of your diaphragm, you will be more in tuned to what your diaphragm is capable of as well as its true limitation.

The voluntary contraction of the diaphragm allows you to generate a slow and long contraction. It allows you to bring the contraction to its absolute limit. Voluntary contraction of the diaphragm not only strengthens your diaphragm but also strengthens your will, as you must have the desire to want to do a full contraction. When you voluntarily engage in a full contraction of the diaphragm, you are giving the body your best effort to supply it with the very vital substance(s) it needs to function to the best of its ability, such as oxygen. You also give the body your best effort in removing the metabolic wastes from it upon full exhalation. Vigorous physical activity involuntarily increases the engagement of the diaphragm out of panic of disruption of homeostasis and to quickly replace what is being lost. Voluntary breathing due to the voluntary contraction of the diaphragm can influence the increase in involuntary breathing from the increase involuntary contraction of the diaphragm from vigorous activity to remain more calm.

After vigorous training of an hour or so, the diaphragm goes back to its normal involuntary breathing rate for the rest of the day, as vigorous physical activity is not performed all day. There is more time spent in sedentary situations where voluntary engagement of the diaphragm proves most beneficial, still providing strength training for the diaphragm and an abundance of oxygen for the body. There is no inspiration without inhalation. In training and strengthening of the diaphragm, all that it requires is for the diaphragm to contract and relax, but the contraction should be full or near a complete contraction, just as what is needed to occur with other skeletal muscles during regular strength training regiments.

Unlike the rapid involuntary contractions of the diaphragm from vigorous physical activity, the contractions from voluntary contraction should be done slowly and gently to a full contraction and sometimes maybe slightly beyond it comfortably (controlled inhalation) and then the relaxation of the diaphragm could also be done slowly and gently (controlled exhalation). The relaxation of the diaphragm also can be allowed to just guide itself following release of the contraction. The way to know that the contraction of the diaphragm is greater than the usual involuntary contraction upon inhalation is by voluntarily inhaling beyond the inhalation point of your normal involuntary inhalation. This would mean that the length of time of inhalation would be longer than the length of time for the involuntary inhalation.

As the diaphragm approaches full or near maximum contraction, it will begin to take more physical effort to continue to inhale and you may feel the diaphragm beginning to pull downward. As a preference, in the beginning, you want the inhalation to be slow to increase the time for oxygen absorption into the blood. You also should inhale through the nose so that the air may be filtered and warmed before entering the lungs. You should inhale until you feel slight tension in the diaphragm. This tension would be felt due to the resistance from the attachment points of the ribs and lumbar spine. You may also inhale until you feel as if you cannot draw in anymore air. Either way, the diaphragm has been contracted beyond its comfort zone or near its contractional limit. At this point, it is 263 time to relax the diaphragm and exhale. You may exhale through the nose or the mouth.

You may let the exhalation guide itself since it is relaxation for the diaphragm and you are removing wastes. It is okay to remove metabolic wastes at a faster rate than the intake of oxygen. You may also control the exhalation for a slow exhalation. This practice should be done standing or sitting, preferably with an erect spine. If done in the standing position, however, be sure to have at least a slight bend in the knees. But it can basically be accomplished in any position. If done lying on the back, the upper body should be slightly elevated above the lower body. Lying flat on the back is fine, too, however. When lying flat on your back you may have your knees bent. Lying on the side is fine.

The advantage of doing this practice standing versus sitting is that when you stand, you have less bends and curves throughout the body, mainly at the knees providing the least resistive pathways for blood to flow and less kinks in the blood vessels. You also can take advantage of gravity pulling blood and fluid into the feet and then using the full contractions of the diaphragm to pull the blood out of the legs, which will then pull blood out of the feet. If need use of the chair anyway, try to sit at the edge as to minimize resistance to blood flow from the pressure of the chair against the hips.

If you choose to stand, you should stand with feet shoulder-width apart, pressing the feet slightly into the floor with the pressure under the feet directed right behind the instep. The knees should be slightly bent, the spine in the thoracic region should be elongated, the spine in the cervical regions should be elongated, ears slightly drawn back, with the chin down if you can. By elongating your spine, you may feel the organs begin the hang.

While sitting in a chair, sit at the edge, knees at 90 degrees, elongate the neck at the thoracic and cervical spine, press ears slightly back and keep chin down. Hands can be placed palms up or down on the knees. Or you may place your hands at your sides. Be sure to hydrate before if you can.

A controlled inhalation should be the focus, as it serves as a greater impact than a controlled exhalation. At the end point of the relaxation of the diaphragm, you can hold it for about two seconds before you begin inhalation, thereby increasing the rest period for the diaphragm. The longer your inhalation or engagement of the diaphragm, the more time you give for this increase of oxygen to enter the body. This practice can be done in just about any sedentary situation such as sitting at a desk, watching TV, working on a computer, talking on the phone, writing a paper, lying down, and even walking. And you do not need a lot of space, so this practice can be performed just about anywhere. If the diaphragm needs rest, then the involuntary contractions will provide that.

Now you can do activities for hours and know that your diaphragm is still getting stronger, contributing to better health. You can't read and jog, but you can read and still exercise your diaphragm. Always listen to your body. Practice times can go from one minute to five minutes to ten minutes to twenty minutes, eventually, to an hour to all day if you can or just whatever time is comfortable for you. You may even count the breaths and do ten full breaths every hour or do one hundred to three hundred full breaths a day as another option. Remember each full breath would be from a voluntary complete/full contraction of the diaphragm. Are you fully engaging your diaphragm now?

The Benefits of the Strengthening of the Diaphragm

Every time you contract the diaphragm, the body pulls in oxygen and chi (as air flows into your body). So the greater you contract your diaphragm using a voluntary diaphragmatic contraction beyond normal involuntary or unconscious diaphragmatic contraction, the deeper and fuller your breath becomes and the longer your inhalation. Therefore, you draw in even more air than a normal involuntary diaphragmatic contraction. The amount of time the air spends in the lungs also becomes longer. This longer inhalation of air brings in more oxygen and more chi with that single breath and allows more time for the oxygen and chi to enter the body than a normal involuntary breath would. As you voluntarily contract the diaphragm to its capacity, you also strengthen the diaphragm. This encourages the development of stronger muscle fibers within the diaphragm. And over time, with continuous practice/training, the diaphragm will contribute toward a positive progression for the capability of an even longer contraction cycle and a substantial further increase in the availability of oxygen for the whole body.

In consequence from just the practice of strengthening the diaphragm alone, you bring in more oxygen and chi, providing more energy and strength for the entire body while reducing stress just by taking an honest full voluntary breath. This would require a full voluntary contraction of the diaphragm. As your diaphragm strengthens over time, each inhalation will draw in even more air, oxygen, and chi in a single breath than the previous. That is unlike the function of the strengthening of any other muscle in the body, as no other muscle brings in oxygen like the diaphragm does. This level of contraction from the diaphragm will also increase blood and fluid circulation in the body. It is necessary to bring in the body more breath, oxygen, and chi than it needs for ordinary function in order to become extraordinary.

Always exhale when you feel the need to with all breathing practices. The evidence of a strengthening/strengthened diaphragm over time would involve the capability of the diaphragm to perform a deeper and lengthier controlled inhalation as well as a well-controlled lengthier exhalation. The measurement of the longer inhalation can be timed. The stronger your diaphragm becomes, the longer your inhalation becomes due to the longer contraction cycle of stronger contracting muscle fibers of the developed diaphragm. A more developed diaphragm is also able to utilize the increase in available oxygen more efficiently with the increased number of mitochondria and capillaries in the muscle fibers of the diaphragm. This is a phenomenon that usually occurs with all skeletal muscles undergoing increased aerobic activity and physical training. This increased aerobic activity for the diaphragm is performed just from a full engagement of the diaphragm. A goal can or may be to work toward being able to give an honest one cycle of an inhalation and an exhalation in the time frame of one minute to five minutes. Or you can quantify it instead and perform up to as many full breaths as you want in a day. The less breaths you take per minute due to lengthier contractions of the diaphragm the better. On average, people take about twelve breaths per minute. Note: If your diaphragm gets tired from numerous voluntary diaphragmatic contractions, then to recover, you can always let the natural involuntary diaphragmatic contractions resume, allowing the involuntary breaths to resume.

As you get better with the training of the diaphragm, you can work on making the contractions of the diaphragm even slower as well as relaxing the diaphragm slower, resulting in even slower breaths. A good practice eventually is to try to infuse both systems together in which you strongly influence engagement of the involuntary diaphragmatic contraction, then take over with the voluntary contraction once the involuntary contraction of the diaphragm reaches its limit, but I will not go into details here.

Believe it or not, a full contraction of the diaphragm alone can help to adjust, improve, and maintain your posture with minimal effort from anything else, as the contraction of the diaphragm opens the rib cage and decompresses the spine by elongating it in the lumbar region, the location where most of the stress in the spine occur. It can also be used to counteract gravity. Anyone interested in guidance or classes for diaphragm strengthening practice should reach out to the author.

In Conclusion

The breath is everything. If you do not have the breath, then you have nothing because without the breath, you could not exist. To access this breath, you must access it through the "power" and function of diaphragm. There is no known limitation as to how strong the diaphragm can be developed and contract, so a good practice would be to attempt to strengthen the diaphragm indefinitely over a lifetime.

In good faith, we should be conscious breathers. This means that at every possible moment, we should make the conscious effort to not only be aware of our breath or breathing but to also take full meaningful breaths with every breath taken. In order to do this, focus should be placed on the diaphragm and the diaphragm should be contracted beyond the contractional effort of its involuntary contraction, preferably to its full/complete capacity. In this way, the control of the breath is maintained and the body can be afforded more input of oxygen if not the maximum input of oxygen possible with every breath taken.

You are the only person that has control over your diaphragm to take advantage of inhaling a full plentiful breath. You are the only one that can make it happen. This process or practice of the development of the diaphragm should continue throughout one's entire life. Would you be willing to practice breathing with full breaths at every possible moment by exercising a full contraction of the diaphragm? Know that the amount of breath entering your body has a direct effect on your life and know that the abundance of oxygen in the body promotes better health and contributes to the prevention of illness. The power is yours; it has always been. It is good faith to make conscientious effort to strengthen, be aware, and fully engage the main skeletal muscle that supports and influences the continuation of life, the diaphragm.

The Diaphragm and The Heart

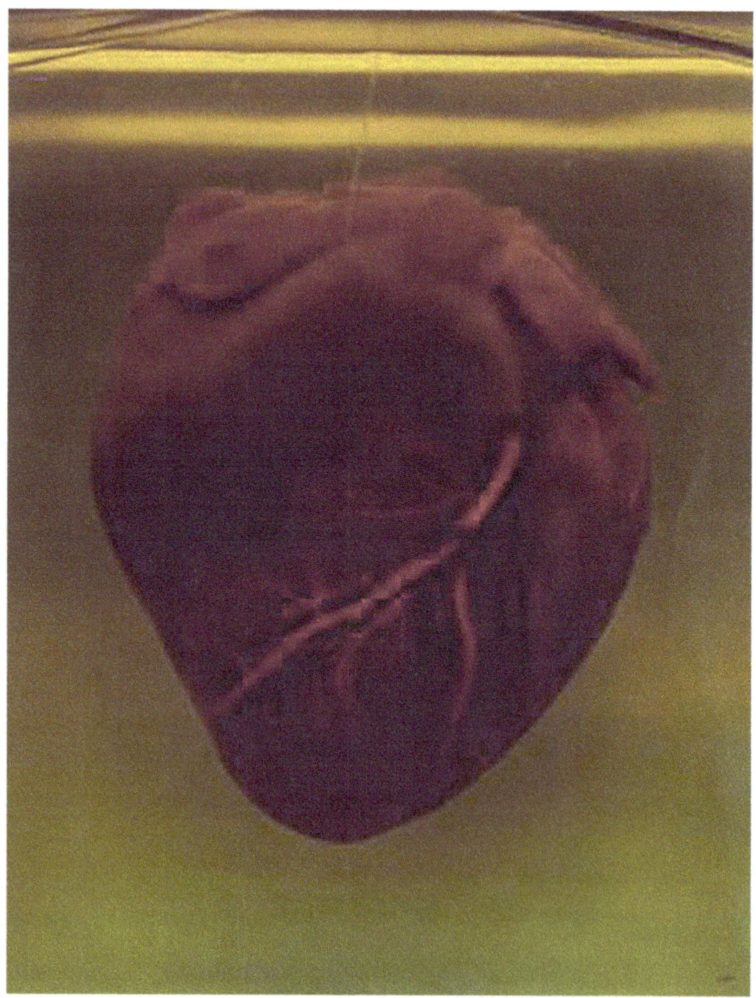

The diaphragm supports heart function.

Introduction

The heart is a muscle that functions autonomously/involuntarily. The involuntary contractions of the heart pumps blood through blood vessels that extend throughout to virtually all the tissues and cells in the body. In contrast to skeletal muscle, cardiac muscle produces little of the ATP or energy it needs by anaerobic respiration (energy-producing reactions that do not require oxygen). Instead, it relies almost exclusively on aerobic respiration (energy-producing reactions that do require oxygen) from its numerous mitochondria. In a person at rest, the heart's ATP/energy comes mainly from oxidation of fatty acids (60 %) and glucose (35 %) with smaller contributions from lactic acid, amino acids, and ketone bodies. During exercise, the heart's use of lactic acid, produced by actively contracting skeletal muscle, rises; however, energy produced from lactic acid (lactate) isn't very much

Just like the diaphragm, if the heart would cease to function, so would life, but in this case, due to the inability of the body to transport oxygenated blood to the whole body. I will digress for a moment. Even though most talk is about healthy heart and lungs, talks should also be turned toward a strong and healthy diaphragm as well, as the diaphragm is multidimensional. The diaphragm is a thick skeletal muscle situated and designed not to tear, can handle stress, and further develops from stress indefinitely like all skeletal muscles, skeletal muscles, in which we have conscious control. Each full contraction of the diaphragm upon inhalation opens the rib cage and elongates the lumbar spine, consequently performing a spinal decompression. This creates more space in the thoracic cavity and supports posture. This improvement in posture contributes to the increase in the potential for maximizing the intake of breath containing vital oxygen, qi/chi, for the increase in blood flow. All this, as a result of the diaphragm's contraction allowing air to enter the body. This improved posture sets up for the increase in the potential as well, on the diaphragm's relaxation upon exhalation, for maximizing the amount of breath containing metabolic wastes and/or turbid qi/chi exiting the body. The diaphragm not only pulls oxygen in on its contraction, but it also aligns and expands the body, putting it into its most efficient position. Now going back to the heart.

Involuntary Control of the Heart

Now the heart beats autonomously, and yes, as it is muscle tissue, it does strengthen when under regular stress from exercise; however, we unfortunately have no direct control over our heart function. Heart function responds to several stimuli, one of them being the levels of carbon dioxide gas (CO_2, or just carbon dioxide) in the blood, most notably when we have a substantial rise in carbon dioxide in the blood. To an extent, the diaphragm function also responds to the levels of carbon dioxide in the blood, notably with rising levels of carbon dioxide as well. As carbon dioxide levels rise substantially in the blood, nerve impulses are sent to both the heart and diaphragm for faster and stronger contractions. Something we experience upon exercising. This response I view as a panic, as the body desperately tries to maintain or restore homeostasis. If carbon dioxide accumulates faster than it is removed, then it is an indication that the oxygen input is not efficient as the volume of the input of oxygen exchanges with the same volume in the removal of carbon dioxide. So if the amount of carbon dioxide accumulates, then there is not a sufficient amount of the input of oxygen to remove a sufficient amount of carbon dioxide. If there is not a sufficient amount of oxygen input then it will be difficult for the body to supply a sufficient amount of energy. If this type of response goes on for too long, it could cause complications with heart function such as a heart attack and/or spasms in the diaphragm if energy expenditure exceeds energy production, as energy is required for the relaxation of the muscle, so that it may contract again. If there is no energy to relax the muscle, then it will remain in stasis.

In addition to bringing in and transporting more oxygen, the increase in the involuntary function of the heart and diaphragm occurs to facilitate the quick removal of carbon dioxide gas from the blood in order to prevent a buildup. An increase in carbon dioxide levels in the blood is linked to the increased production of acids, so a buildup of carbon dioxide gas in the blood would contribute to an increase in acidity in the blood in addition to lactic acid released from muscles. This increase in the production of acids would increase the acidity of the blood as the body tries to keep the blood in an alkaline state. This increase in the acidity of the blood could lower the pH of the blood. As the blood becomes more acidic, the red blood cells, which are the cells that carry the oxygen, become less capable of holding on to this precious oxygen, decreasing the availability of oxygen for particular parts of the body. Fortunately, the increase in the delivery of oxygen has the capability of reducing lactic acid levels.

The optimal pH for the blood is between 7.35 and 7.45. This range is considered the alkaline range. This creates an optical environment for cellular enzyme activity and membrane integrity. The body uses energy to maintain this pH range. The energy made available to try and maintain this pH range is supported by the availability of oxygen. So on one hand, with rapid heartbeat and breathing due to increasing levels of carbon dioxide, oxygen is quickly being drawn in to provide the energy to maintain the blood's pH range of 7.35 through 7.45. And on the other hand, the body is rapidly removing carbon dioxide gas, which would reduce the accumulation of acid production.

Voluntary Contraction of the Diaphragm and Heart Activity

Even though there is an increase in the involuntary activity of the heart and diaphragm in response to nerve impulses when there is an increase in carbon dioxide in the blood, voluntary control of the diaphragm is still possible. If we deeply consciously inhale by means of a complete or maximum contraction of the diaphragm and deeply exhale consciously by means of a complete relaxation of the diaphragm with every breath we take, we can maintain lower levels of carbon dioxide in the blood and higher oxygen levels in the blood, even during exercise or any level of physical exertion. This can prevent the heart contractions from becoming excessively rapid. The heart can then continue to beat or function more peacefully but effectively when the diaphragm takes the wheel. This would also prevent the diaphragm from going into a panic that we view as a breathing panic, in which we are then instructed to regain control of our breathing by breathing.

I say you should take control over your diaphragm in order to control your breathing. Reminder, full voluntary contraction of the diaphragm allows for the relative maximum entry of oxygen into the body at the same time it allows for the relative maximum amount of carbon dioxide to be released upon its full relaxation.

The Four Chambers of the Heart (Right Atrium, Left Atrium, Right Ventricle, Left Ventricle)

During the contraction cycle of the heart, it relatively begins in the right border of the heart called the right atrium. This is where deoxygenated blood (blood without oxygen) is received from the entire body through three veins: the superior vena cava, the inferior vena cava, and the coronary sinus. The superior vena cava returns deoxygenated blood to the heart from the systemic circulation of the upper half of the body above the diaphragm. The inferior vena cava returns deoxygenated blood to the heart from the systemic circulation of the middle and lower half of the body below the diaphragm. And the coronary sinus returns deoxygenated blood to the heart from the systemic circulation of the great, middle, small, and anterior veins of the heart.

Upon receiving this deoxygenated blood, the right atrium will then contract and send this deoxygenated blood into the right ventricle. The right ventricle will then contract and send the deoxygenated blood to the pulmonary trunk (lungs), this is the location where the blood is oxygenated. The left atrium then receives this oxygenated blood from the pulmonary trunk (lungs). The left atrium will then contract and send the oxygenated blood to the left ventricle. The left ventricle will then contract and eject the oxygenated blood to the rest of the body. The two atria contract simultaneously while the two ventricles are relaxed. The two ventricles then contract simultaneously while the two atria are relaxed. Then all four chambers, the two atria and two ventricles, briefly remain relaxed simultaneously.

Stroke Volume

Now I want to talk about something with the heart called the stroke volume. The stroke volume is the amount of blood that is ejected from the heart through ventricular contraction. There are two ventricles, right and left. The significance of ventricular contraction is that one ventricle sends deoxygenated blood to receive oxygen from the lungs and the other ventricle sends the oxygenated blood to the rest of the body. Both ventricles eject the same volume of blood upon simultaneous contraction.

Now a healthy heart will pump out the volume of blood that entered its chambers during the previous resting period (diastole). So then if a greater volume of venous blood returns to the heart during the resting period, then that greater volume of blood will be ejected from the heart during the contraction period (systole). The reason for this is that when more blood fills the heart during the resting period, this increase in the volume of blood causes a greater degree of stretching within the muscle fibers of the heart.

This increase, in the stretching of the muscle fibers of the heart during the resting period, stimulates an increase in force of contraction by the heart generated on the blood by the heart, ejecting more blood to the body per contraction from the heart. This action allows the heart to stay true in its function to support "what you put in is what you get out." So the ejection of this increased amount of blood would contribute to a considerable increase in stroke volume. Simply put, this means that this ejection of more blood per contraction would contribute to a considerable increase in blood circulation.

It is known that a lot of heath—mental, physical, and emotional—problems can begin with poor circulation. Poor circulation means less oxygen availability, less availability of nutrients, as well as less removal of metabolic wastes and energy production. So an increase in stroke volume from the heart may improve these conditions, as the right atrium is connected to the largest veins in the body, and the left ventricle is connected to the largest artery (aorta) in the body, creating the potential for a substantial increase in stroke volume. This arrangement demonstrates just how equipped and capable the heart is in receiving a substantial volume of blood and ejecting a substantial or large volume of blood.

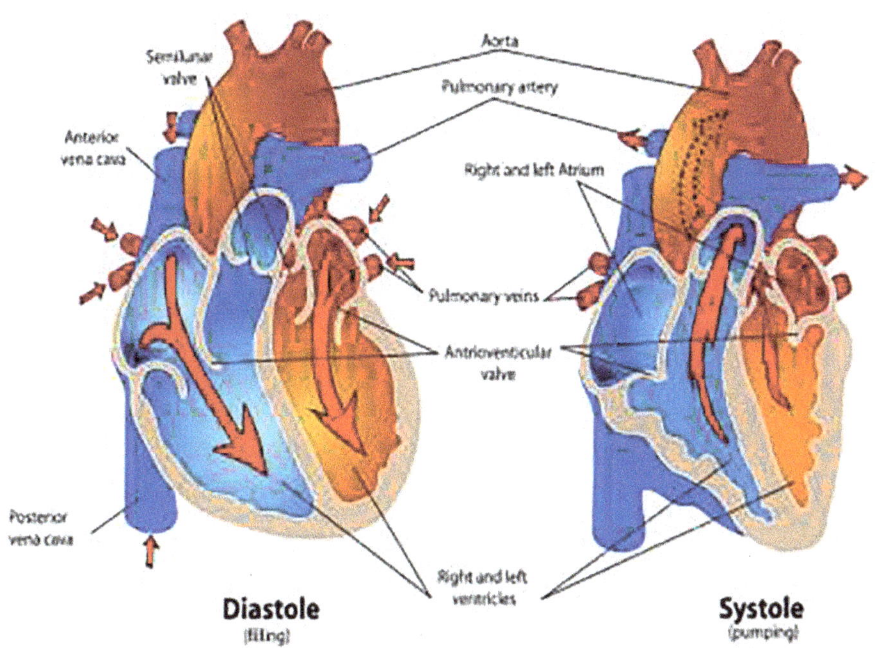
Aorta
Semilunar valve
Pulmonary artery
Anterior vena cava
Right and left Atrium
Pulmonary veins
Antrioventicular valve
Posterior vena cava
Right and left ventricles
Diastole
(filing)
Systole
(pumping)

The Diaphragm's Contribution to the Increase in Stroke Volume

I would now like to discuss two factors that contribute to an increase in stroke volume (circulation). Both factors allow an increase in the amount of venous blood to return to the heart during its resting period and before the heart's next "ventricular" contraction.

Factor 1 refers to the length of time that the ventricles remain at rest before contraction. This factor states that the longer the length of time that the ventricles remain at rest before their next contraction, the longer the length of time the ventricles have to fill with blood before their next contraction. So then the longer the ventricles stay relaxed the, the more time it has to fill up with blood before it contracts.

Factor 2 involves the volume of the venous blood that is received by the right ventricle because of the volume of venous blood returned to the right atrium. This factor states that if you increase the volume of venous blood that returns to the right atrium before the contraction of the right atrium, then you will increase the volume of blood received by the right ventricle before ventricular contraction. The blood volume pumped by the right ventricle is dependent upon the volume received by the right atrium. So by increasing the time between ventricular contractions (factor 1) and by increasing atrial blood volume (factor 2) you can effectively increase stroke volume or blood circulation.

The function of the diaphragm can positively influence these two factors. Therefore, the responsibility should 496 be placed if not heavily placed on the diaphragm to help the heart increase blood circulation. Support of factor 1 would require the heart rate to decrease. A decrease in heart rate would provide longer rest periods between contractions. One way to indirectly accomplish this would be to keep carbon dioxide levels low in the blood. As stated before, the harder the diaphragm works by continuous voluntary, conscious, full contractions and relaxations, the input of oxygen increases and the removal of carbon dioxide also increases, lowering the amount of carbon dioxide in the blood. This will result in the nervous system to influence the heart rate to slowdown. As a result, the heart will beat at its slowest possible rate relative to its own fitness level, increasing the length of time between the ventricular contractions. This allows more time for venous blood to fill the ventricles before the next ventricular contraction. This extra time would then lead to an increase in the volume of venous blood received by the ventricles before the next ventricular contraction, increasing stroke volume (circulation). As the heart functions under less stressful conditions, its energy expenditure decreases, and its function becomes more efficient.

The factor that states that "the greater the volume of venous blood returned to the right atrium before the contraction of the right atrium results in a greater volume of blood received by the right ventricle before ventricular contraction" would require an increase in the amount or volume of blood to return to the heart. Since veins are the blood vessels that returns blood to the heart, then actions that stimulate more blood to flow through the veins would be necessary such as muscle contractions. Each voluntary, conscious, full contraction of the diaphragm pushes a greater amount of blood back to the heart.

To get a little technical, the increased voluntary, conscious contraction of the diaphragm (deep inhalation) causes a greater amount of blood to move from abdominal veins (vena cava) by the increase in compression on them into the decompressed thoracic veins and then into the right atrium before its contraction. This increase in the the blood volume returned to the heart will be ejected by the heart during ventricular contraction. This action supports factor 2 previously mentioned for an increase in stroke volume (circulation). When the pressures reverse during the relaxation of the diaphragm (exhalation), the valves in the veins prevent backflow of the blood from the thoracic veins to the abdominal veins until the next contraction of the diaphragm. This is considered a milking action. The other skeletal muscles also do participate in this milking action when they are active in support of venous blood return, but the diaphragm does it closer to the heart and is constantly functioning and has access to a significant volume of blood.

In conclusion, if a more conscientious effort is put into the contraction and relaxation of the diaphragm, then less stress will be placed on the heart, allowing the heart to beat or function at a slower (calmer), more peaceful rate, possibly reducing the risk or onset of heart complications while increasing circulation for the whole body. Simply put, maximizing the function of the diaphragm maximizes oxygen input and carbon dioxide output, which maximizes the efficiency of the function of the lungs, which leads to maximizing the efficiency of the heart as this leads to the eventual rate of the heartbeat to slow down.

With the heart rate slowed down, each resting period of the heart allows for the increased input of blood. This increased input of blood will then lead to an increase in the stretching of the muscle fibers of the heart. This increase in the stretching of the muscle fibers of the heart will lead to the generation of an increase in the force of contraction by the heart muscle fibers. This increase in the force of contraction from the heart muscles fibers will increase the output of blood by the heart. This action ensures that the volume of blood received by the heart will always be pumped out by the heart. The action of increasing the force of contraction by the heart from the increase in blood return for the heart tends to strengthen the heart in the process.

On another note, maximizing the function of the diaphragm maximizes the return of venous blood to the heart, supporting factor 2. This also contributes to the increase in the stretching of and force of contraction by the heart muscle fibers. If the diaphragm takes care of the heart, then the heart can and will take care of the body.

Note: Increasing the volume of venous blood that is returned to the heart per beat results in a more forceful contraction of the heart muscles in order to eject that increased volume of blood. This increase in blood volume comes from an increase in atrial blood volume. The ejection of this increased volume of atrial blood from the left ventricle is key to activating parasympathetic nerve activity.

The Diaphragm Gives the Heart a Purpose

Let us be clear. The function of the heart is to contract. Its contraction is designed to create a flow of blood that travels in one direction throughout the body. The blood leaves the heart from one blood vessel and returns to the heart through another blood vessel; therefore, the heart beats to perform this task. For this flow of blood to be beneficial, the blood needs to carry oxygen, in addition to nutrients, so that a continuous supply of oxygen may be transported and delivered throughout the body. As the heart pumps blood, the blood is directed through the lungs, where it picks up the oxygen that is needed throughout the body. Both the heart and lungs work in conjunction with the function of the diaphragm as the contraction of the diaphragm ensures the return of venous blood to the heart and simultaneously provides the oxygen in the lungs to be picked up by that same blood.

Some limitation of the heart

As the heart transports blood carrying oxygen around the body, the cells of the heart use oxygen for energy. Yet the heart itself cannot replenish the oxygen for itself or for the rest of the body alone but only in conjunction with the diaphragm. Consequently, the waste products generated by the heart from its own energy production must also be removed from the body, and this responsibility falls on the diaphragm. This removal of waste is accomplished by the exhalation of the lungs as the diaphragm relaxes. This idea supports that the diaphragm keeps the the heart going. In another concept, the heart does help create the lymphatic fluid, and it is the diaphragm that circulates it through the lymphatic system.

A very interesting concept about the diaphragm I would like to mention

Upon contraction of the diaphragm, unusual behavior between air and liquid occurs, as air normally rises and liquids normally fall, but when the diaphragm contracts, the opposite happens. When the diaphragm contracts, liquid in blood flows up into the heart and air flows down into the lungs so that the heart can mix the blood with oxygen.

Now listen to this. I mentioned before that the diaphragm could be voluntarily strengthened. To voluntarily strengthen the diaphragm, the contraction of the diaphragm needs to go beyond the normal involuntary contraction of the diaphragm. This would result in a bigger breath taken. When this increase in contraction of the diaphragm occurs, there would be an increase in the volume of blood returned to the heart during its the resting period. This increase in the volume of blood would increase the stretching of the heart muscle fibers. This increase in the stretching of the heart muscle fibers would stimulate a stronger contraction by the heart muscle. Along with adequate oxygen input, these stronger contractions exercise the heart, making it stronger. So then by increasing the heart's venous blood return may result in the strengthening of the heart, which would then come from voluntarily strengthening diaphragm alone as opposed to only involuntarily increasing the heart's rate or frequency of contraction from regular exercise. So look at that, you can strengthen your heart just by voluntarily strengthening your diaphragm, and it can be done while you are watching TV, reading my book, or typing a paper. You can't beat that!

Comparison between the Diaphragm and the Heart

The heart must be able to coordinate between four chambers to effectively direct the flow of blood around the body in one direction. Any disruption to this coordination can create a backflow of blood, which should be unidirectional, hindering adequate blood flow and delaying oxygen and nutrient delivery, as well as waste removal.

The overall function of the diaphragm is much simpler than the function of the heart. It does not require complicated coordination. The simple function of the diaphragm makes it difficult for the diaphragm to disrupt the flow and delivery of blood. It also makes it difficult for the diaphragm to disrupt the flow of air entering and exiting the body. This allows the diaphragm to able to maintain the consistent availability of oxygen and the consistent removal of carbon dioxide. Due to this, it makes sense to increase engagement of the diaphragm at times, as it can help maintain integrity of heart function.

Once again, it does not require strenuous exercise to strengthen the diaphragm. There are practices that take more of a mental focus with just a little physical effort instead in order to strengthen the diaphragm. Therefore, the opportunities for diaphragm training or strengthening maybe almost limitless, as it can be, once again, done while watching TV, going for a walk, driving, while stuck in traffic, in the hospital, recovering from COVID-19, or while doing almost any activity. When a full, conscious, voluntary contraction of the diaphragm is achieved, then diaphragm strengthening is occurring. Basically, if you are awake, then the opportunity is there.

The Diaphragm and Belly Breathing

Belly breathing is a known form of breathing where the focus on the breathing is to push the stomach out as you inhale. Even so, the diaphragm is still required to perform belly breathing. No matter how far you push your belly out, the limit of taking in breath is dependent on the contractional limit of the diaphragm. If you just focus on the diaphragm and do a full contraction of the diaphragm, then the breath is maximized whether you push the stomach out or not.

The Diaphragm and The Lungs

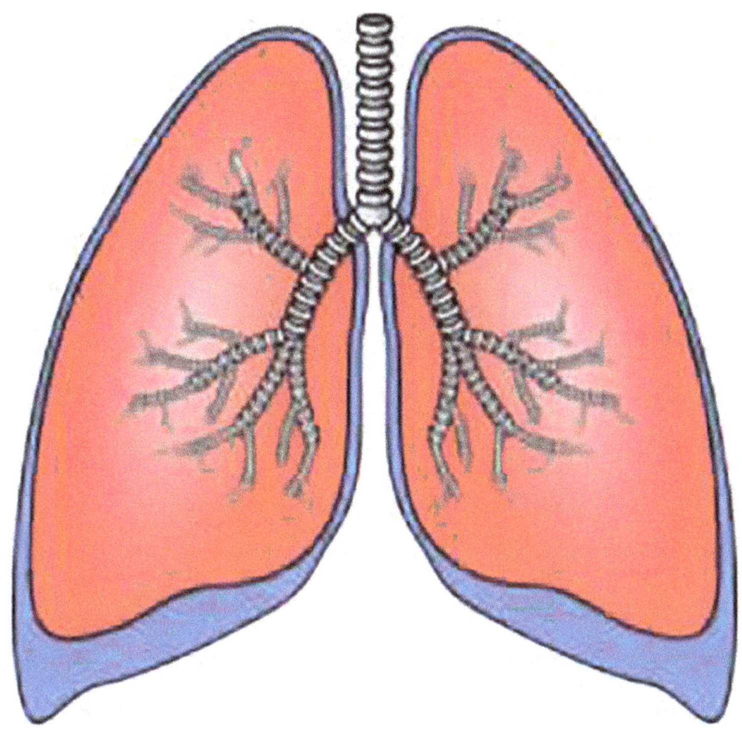

The diaphragm supports lung function.

The known importance of the function of the lungs is to transfer life-giving oxygen into the blood as well as receive/remove metabolic wastes such as carbon dioxide from the blood. The production of carbon dioxide is a consequence of life-preserving energy production. This process of energy production is called cellular respiration or cellular metabolism. Once carbon dioxide is removed from the blood into lungs, it must then be expunged from the lungs out of the body. Before oxygen can become available in the lungs for transfer, oxygen must enter the lungs. In order for oxygen to flow into the lungs, the diaphragm must contract. If the diaphragm does not contract, then the air or breath that carries oxygen and chi will not flow into the lungs. This would prevent the lungs from providing the blood with fresh oxygen.

On the other hand, once the lungs collect the carbon dioxide from the blood, the lungs must then release it from the body. Before the carbon dioxide collected in lungs can be released from the body, the diaphragm must relax. If the diaphragm does not relax, then the lungs would be unable to recoil and push the carbon dioxide out of the body.

Therefore, it is the diaphragm that is responsible for the inhalation of the oxygen that flows into the lungs that would be available to enter the blood. The diaphragm is also responsible for the exhalation of carbon dioxide from the lungs received by the blood. This indicates that lung function is related to diaphragm function as lung function is dependent upon the physical effects from the diaphragm. The expansion of the lungs is dictated by the degree of contraction of the diaphragm. The more the diaphragm is contracted, the more the lungs expand. The more the diaphragm is relaxed, the more the lungs contract. That is how the lungs get exercise, repetitious contraction and relaxation of the diaphragm.

The Diaphragm Influences the Lungs

Also, in situations where breathing appears to be impaired, focus should not be placed on only the lungs but also on the diaphragm. The function of the diaphragm can move and change the shape of the lungs during its contraction and relaxation cycle, contributing to the constant pumping action of the lungs. This could possibly prevent the settling of particles in the lungs that could interfere with the proper functioning of the lungs such as microbes, viruses, or other foreign material. Forceful exhalations of the diaphragm can effectively purge the lungs. When tissues in the body are not effectively stretched, they can get tight over time, preventing healthy movement and fluid flow.

Full expansion and contraction of the lungs is the best care you can give to the lungs to keep them clear and healthy aided by the full engagement of the diaphragm. This would require voluntary, conscious control. You would also be filling the lungs to capacity with oxygen that would also be beneficial to the lungs. We should always try our best, when possible, to maximize our breath intake, as the breath is just about the strongest form of protection and support for the lungs.

The Diaphragm and The Brain

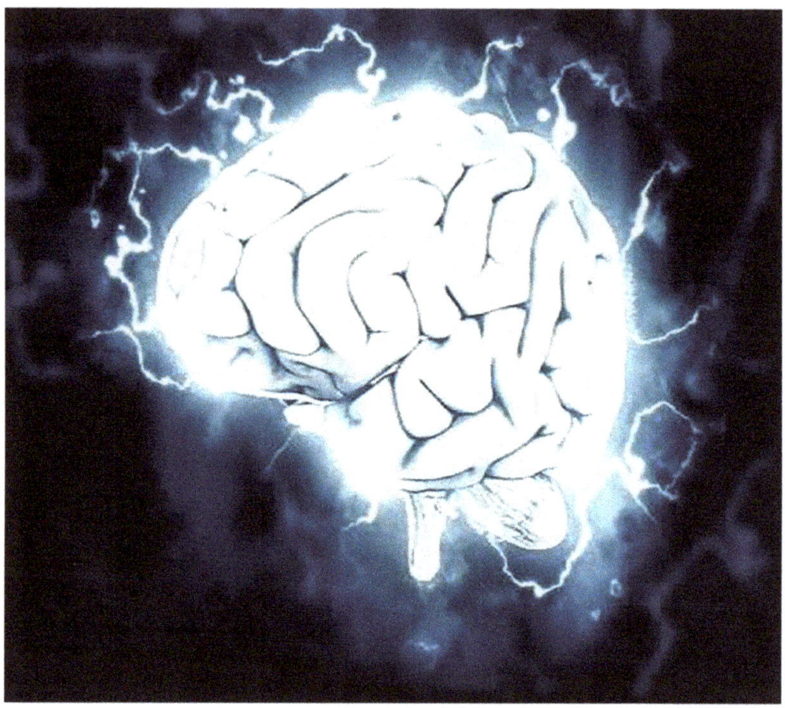

The diaphragm regulates the functional level of the brain.

The brain is an organ that serves as the center of the nervous system in humans. It is located in the head, close to the sensory organs of the senses such as vision. It is the most complex organ in our body. The function of the brain interprets information from the outside world and embodies the essence of the mind and soul. The brain controls our thoughts, memory, and speech; movement of the arms and legs; and the function of many organs within our body. When it comes to the metabolism of the brain, the brain consumes up to 20 % of the energy used by the human body, more than any other organ. In an adult, the brain represents 2 % of total body weight but consumes about 20 % of the total oxygen consumption and 20 % to 25 % of the total glucose used, even at rest, and receives 15 % of the cardiac output.

Neurons (brain cells) synthesize ATP (energy) almost exclusively from glucose via reactions with oxygen. When glucose levels are low, the brain can use other compounds for energy such as ketone bodies (from oxidation of fatty acids), fatty acids (small, medium), and lactate (from lactic acid created during exercise by glycolysis without the presence of oxygen). These compounds are more abundant in the bloodstream during those times glucose levels are low, in which each of those compounds require oxygen for complete metabolism. Complete metabolism will provide the maximum amount of energy possible. This adaptive capability by the brain ensures and maintains a continuous source of energy for the brain.

When the activity of the neurons and neuroglia increases in a region of the brain, blood flow to that area also increases. Blood flow to the brain is very vital as even a brief slowing of the brain's blood flow may cause unconsciousness. Typically, an interruption in blood flow for one to two minutes impairs neuronal function, and total deprivation of oxygen for about four minutes causes permanent injury.

Because virtually no glucose is stored in the brain, supply of glucose must be continuous. If blood entering the brain has a low level of glucose, mental confusion, dizziness, convulsions, and loss of consciousness may occur. Be as it is stated that total deprivation of oxygen for four minutes (which is relatively a short amount of time) causes permanent injury reinforces just how important constant oxygen availability is to the brain, indicating just how crucial the constant production of energy (ATP) is to the brain as well as the continuous flow of blood since it is the blood that delivers the oxygen and glucose needed for energy production.

There is no major storage system of oxygen as we see in the likes of food and water; therefore, we need a constant ready supply of oxygen. The muscle in the body that is responsible for this constant availability of oxygen is the diaphragm. The amount of effort placed on the diaphragm's contraction can determine what abundance of oxygen the brain can and will receive. With the brain being the most complex organ, it consumes more of the total energy than any other organ in the body. The more energy the brain has access to, then the more efficient it should function. The availability of energy for the brain is directly related to the availability of oxygen for the brain since maximizing the output of energy from the energy-producing reactions involving the brain require oxygen. It seems to compliment well with the relationship that the more you contract your diaphragm, the more oxygen you make available for your body. When more oxygen becomes available for your body, then more oxygen becomes available for your brain. When more oxygen becomes available for your brain, then more energy becomes available for your brain. When more energy becomes available for your brain, then your brain will increase in function and development. Can I say the diaphragm equals brain function, or more diaphragm equals more brain function, or less diaphragm equals less brain function?

In conclusion, the more effort you put into the function of your diaphragm, the more effort you get out of the function of your brain.

The Diaphragm and Cerebral Spinal Fluid

On this last note, I would like to briefly discuss the diaphragm and its role with cerebral spinal fluid. Cerebral spinal fluid (CSF) is a clear, colorless fluid found in the brain and spinal cord. And its role is to protect the brain and spinal cord from trauma, supply nutrients to nervous system tissue, and remove waste products from cerebral metabolism. It has been concluded that this fluid is pumped every time you take a breath in or upon inhalation. Upon inhalation, the sacrum rocks backward along with the cervical spine, and on the exhalation, the sacrum rocks forward along with the cervical spine. This pattern induces a rhythmic pulse at the base of the spine and base of the skull that pumps the fluid circulating in the spinal canal and brain

Inhalation is controlled by the diaphragm, indicating that the diaphragm has influence over the amount of cerebral spinal fluid that is pumped. It is the diaphragm that rocks the sacrum and cervical spine backward and forward upon its contraction and relaxation cycles. The increase in the conscious, voluntary engagement of the diaphragm will generate an increase in the amount of CSF that will be pumped.

Effects of Aging on the Nervous System

When it comes to aging and the nervous system, from early adulthood onward, brain mass declines. By the time a person reaches eighty, the brain weighs about 7 % less than it did in young adulthood. Although the number of neurons present does not decrease very much, the number of synaptic contacts declines. Associated with the decrease in brain mass is a decreased capacity for sending nerve impulses to and from the brain. As a result, processing of information diminishes, conduction velocity decreases, voluntary motor movements slow down, and reflex times increase.

Just as many things decline as you age, physical activity declines and muscles that are not exercised weaken. When physical activity declines and we only allow the autonomic nervous system to breathe for us, it does not influence the maximum contraction or full contraction of the diaphragm; therefore, the amount of oxygen taken into the body is not maximized. This reduction of oxygen intake reduces the total amount of available oxygen for the body as well as the brain.

As oxygen levels in the body decreases, so does oxygen levels in the brain, thereby negatively affecting the amount of energy the brain can provide for itself. As energy levels in the brain decrease, so may the function of the brain. Increasing diaphragm function with voluntary diaphragmatic contraction may prove beneficial and continue to support effective brain function.

The Diaphragm and the Kidneys (TCM)

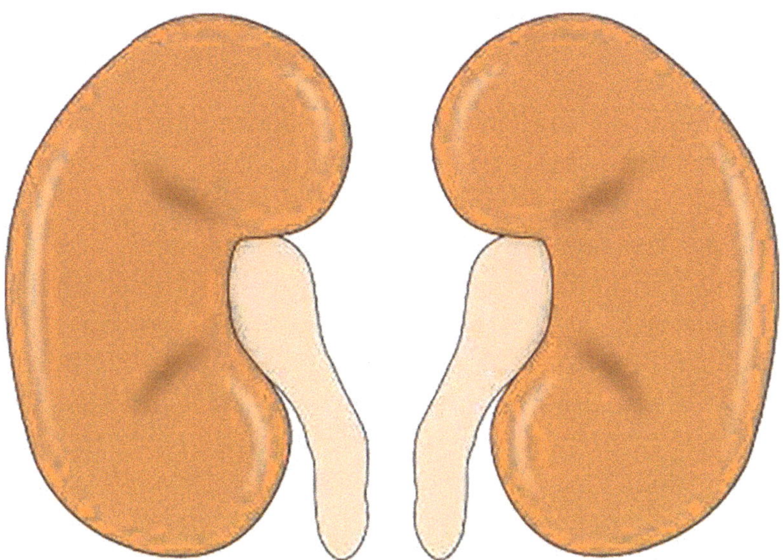

Essence gives the idea of something derived from a process of refinement or distillation. In traditional Chinese medicine (TCM), when a human is conceived, it is achieved from the blending of the sexual energies of man and woman. This forms what the ancient Chinese called the pre-heaven essence (prenatal essence) of the newly conceived human being. This essence nourishes the embryo and fetus during pregnancy and is also dependent upon nourishment derived from the mother's kidneys. The pre-heaven essence is the only kind of essence present in the fetus, as it does not have independent physiological activity. This pre-heaven essence is what determines each person's basic constitutional makeup, strength, and vitality. It is what makes each individual unique. The pre-heaven essence "matures" into kidney essence during puberty.

Since it is inherited from the parents at conception, the pre-heaven essence can be influenced only with difficulty in the course of adult life. Some say this essence is "fixed" in quantity and quality. However, due to its interaction with the post-heaven essence (essence that is refined and extracted from food and fluids by the stomach and spleen after birth), it can be positively affected, even if not quantitatively increased. The best way to positively affect one's pre-heaven essence is by striving for balance in one's life activities: balance between work and rest, restraint in sexual activity, and maintenance of a balanced diet. Any irregularity or excess in these spheres is bound 730 to diminish the pre-heaven essence.

A direct way to influence one's essence positively is through breathing exercises as tai ji quan and qi gong. This concept of breathing exercises falls right in line with diaphragmatic activity. Qi gong translates to breath work or energy work. This energy called qi/chi is believed to enter the body by breathing or inhaling. It can then be further transformed and manipulated to flow in the body through body movements. The more plentiful the breath, then the more energy provided in that breath that can then be used in order to strengthen the pre-heaven essence. It does not only strengthen pre-heaven essence but also never tap into it by providing an abundance of qi/chi in the body.

The practice of generating a full contraction of the diaphragm per breath should be strongly encouraged since that would maximize the breath, providing maximum energy in that breath. This practice should be continued as a way of life with an additional focus on strengthening the diaphragm indefinitely along the life of the practitioner. Indefinitely strengthening the diaphragm can contribute to indefinitely strengthening one's pre-heaven essence by indefinitely increasing one's input of qi/chi, giving the less fortunate a fair shake at life regardless of the parents' energetic input. It is believed that once pre-heaven essence is depleted, then life ends.

The Diaphragm and the Kidneys (Western Medicine)

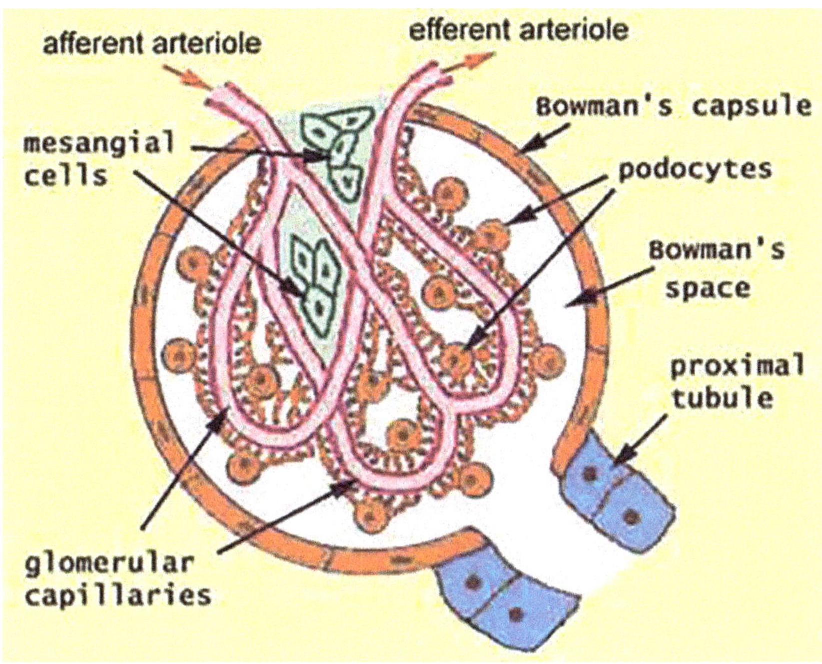

The function of the thoracic diaphragm has the potential and capability of increasing the function of the kidneys by way of the heart.

Introduction

The kidneys are paired, reddish, kidney-bean-shaped organs located just above the waist between the peritoneum and posterior wall of abdomen. Each of the adult size of the kidney is about the size of a bar of soap and has a mass of 135 through 150 grams. Although the kidneys constitute less than 0.5 % of total body mass, they receive 20 through 25 % of the resting cardiac output. In adults, the blood flow through both kidneys (renal blood flow) is about 1,200 milliliters per minute.

The functions of the kidneys include **(1)** regulation of blood ionic composition, **(2)** regulation of blood pH, **(3)** regulation of blood volume, **(4)** regulation of blood pressure, **(5)** maintenance of blood osmolarity, **(6)** production of hormones, **(7)** regulation of blood glucose level, and **(8)** excretion of wastes and foreign substances.

Since the very familiar function of the kidneys is the formation of urine, I would like to go into a little more detail about the necessity of the formation of urine. As the formation of urine is necessary for waste removal and/or pH regulation. By forming urine, the kidneys help excrete wastes substances that have no useful function in the body and may compete with energy production in the body. Some wastes excreted in urine result from metabolic reactions in the body. These include ammonia and urea (from proteins), bilirubin (from red blood cells), creatinine, and uric acid (from DNA, RNA). Other wastes excreted in urine are foreign substances from the diet, such as drugs and environmental toxins. The kidneys also excrete a variable amount of hydrogen ions (H^+), which are acidic, into the urine while conserving bicarbonate ions (HCO_3^-), which are an important buffer of H^+ in the blood. Both of these activities help regulate blood pH; therefore, it is very beneficial to have good kidney function for good health.

A nephron is the functional unit of the kidney in which there are millions. Each nephron consists of two parts: a *renal corpuscle*, where blood plasma (water potion of the blood containing dissolved solutes) is filtered from the blood, and a *renal tubule*, a structure in which the filtered fluid passes. The two components of the renal corpuscle are the glomerulus (capillary network) or glomerular capillaries and the glomerular capsule, a capsule that surrounds the glomerular capillaries. Blood first enters the glomerular capsule through an afferent arteriole, gets filtered, then leaves the glomerular capsule through an efferent arteriole. Blood plasma is filtered from the blood in the glomerular capsule by the glomerular capillaries. This filtered fluid enters the capsule's space and then passes into the renal tubule to be processed. This fluid to be processed. This fluid to be processed later forms urine to be excreted. The focus in this section will be on therenal corpuscle with respect to urine formation.

Filtration of the Kidneys

Glomerular filtration is the first step in urine production, as the blood must be filtered first in the renal corpuscles of kidneys before urine can be formed. The amount of filtrate formed in all the "renal corpuscles" of both kidneys each minute is the glomerular filtration rate (GFR). The rate of filtration can vary; however, the faster the filtration rate, the faster wastes are removed from the blood and the faster the blood is balanced, leading to improved health. The increase in the GFR indicates a more efficient kidney function.

There are two ways to increase the GFR. One way is by increasing the blood flow to the kidneys by lowering blood pressure. The other way is by increasing the surface area of the glomerular capillaries. The surface area of the glomerular capillaries is regulated by mesangial cells. When the mesangial cells are contracted, the surface area of the glomerular capillaries is reduced. When the mesangial cells are relaxed, the surface area of the glomerular capillaries is maximized and glomerular filtration is very high.

An issue with only increasing blood flow to increase GFR is that the limitation of filtration capabilities of the kidneys is dependent upon the amount of the surface area available from the glomerular capillaries. So I will focus on the glomerular capillaries as an effective way for increasing the GFR.

The most effective way however, to increase and maximize the filtration rate in the kidneys would be to maximize the surface area of the glomerular capillaries. In order to do so, the mesangial cells of the glomerular capillaries must be relaxed. For the mesangial cells to function in a relaxed state, they must be stimulated by the hormone atrial natriuretic peptide or ANP. This hormone acts on the kidneys to relax the mesangial cells, maximizing the surface area of the glomerular capillaries and this hormone is released by the heart.

Atrial Natriuretic Peptide

Breaking the words down, "atrial" is referring to the atria of the heart. The right atrium of the heart, one of the four chambers of the heart, is the chamber that receives venous blood return from the superior vena cava, inferior vena cava, and coronary sinus. The left atrium, another of the four chambers of the heart, receives that same blood after it is oxygenated from pulmonary veins. The word "natriuretic" broken down. The "natri" part of the word means salt, "uretic" relates to uresis or excretion, and "peptide" is a small protein. So the atrial natriuretic peptide is a small protein released from the heart cells of the right atrium that relates to salt excretion and relaxes the mesangial cells, maximizing the surface area of the glomerular capillaries. This leads to an increase in the kidney filtration rate or GFR.

This maximizing of the surface area of the glomerular capillaries is what makes the function of the kidneys more efficient. When this peptide (ANP) is not present, the mesangial cells remain in a contracted state, decreasing the surface area of the glomerular capillaries, leading to a decrease in the glomerular filtration rate. This prevents the kidneys from being able to filter or remove necessary substances (excess ions, acids, wastes, toxins) from the blood at its most optimal rate or capability.

The Stimulus for ANP Release

Atrial natriuretic peptide or ANP is released by the cells of the right atrium. The stimulus that influences the muscle cells of the right atrium to release atrial natriuretic peptide (ANP) is from an increase in the stretching of the atrial wall due to increased atrial blood volume. Cells in the atria of the heart contain volume receptors, which respond to increased stretching of the atrial wall due to the increase in the stretching of the atrial wall due to the increase in atrial blood volume. The atria (plural) receive the blood that returns to the heart through the veins. This means that the increase in atrial blood volume could only come from venous blood flow.

The right atrium is the first section of the heat that receives venous blood. The volume of blood received by the right atrium will be pumped to the left atrium through pulmonary veins. So the increase in atrial blood volume is dependent upon the increased blood volume that occurs in the right atrium via the systemic veins known as the super vena cava, inferior vena cava, and coronary sinus.

If the volume of blood returned to the right atrium is enough to cause a greater stretch of the muscle fibers in the right atrium, it will also cause a greater stretch in the muscle fibers of the left atrium. The diaphragm can increase this atrial blood volume for the right atrium through its effect on the blood of the veins that attach to the right atrium, the inferior vena cava, the superior vena cava, and coronary sinus, thus causing the atrial stretch necessary to trigger the release of atrial natriuretic peptide (ANP).

The Diaphragm and the Stimulation of ANP Release

When you engage a voluntary maximum or full contraction of the diaphragm or a contraction of the diaphragm that exceeds the involuntary contraction of the diaphragm, it increases compression on the inferior vena cava, pushing more blood up into the right atrium, increasing the volume of blood entering the right atrium. The maximum or full contraction of the diaphragm also increases the compression on the thoracic duct, which is the largest lymphatic vessel in the body. This greater compression pushes more lymphatic fluid out of the thoracic duct and back into the bloodstream at the junction of the left internal jugular vein and left subclavian vein (left side of your neck). This lymphatic fluid then returns to the right atrium via the superior vena cava.

The combination of the increased volume of blood from the inferior vena cava and the increased volume of lymphatic fluid from the superior vena cava returning to the right atrium of the heart increases atrial blood volume. This increase in atrial blood volume increases the stretching of the atrial walls, as the left atrium will receive the same increased blood volume received by the right atrium. This increase in atrial blood volume will stimulate the cells of the right atrium to release the hormone atrial natriuretic peptide (ANP). Atrial natriuretic peptide will then act on the kidneys to increase their filtration rate, stimulating the kidneys to become more efficient.

Summary

A full or maximum contraction of the diaphragm increases the volume of blood and fluid that returns to the heart by the blood in the veins and the fluid throughout the lymphatic system. This causes the increase in atrial blood volume, which will then increase the heart's stroke volume, which will increase blood circulation. This makes the heart function more efficiently. When the heart functions more efficiently, it then stimulates the kidneys to function more efficiently. Making the function of the heart more efficient leads to making the function of the kidneys more efficient.

I would like to discuss "diaphragmatic breathing" or "deep breathing" commonly used in yoga and qi gong / chi kung practice, as I am a practitioner of both. Not only do you increase the input of oxygen and increase the output of carbon dioxide, which is an increase in the efficiency of the function of the lungs, but it also leads to the increase in the efficiency of the function of the heart, which then leads to the increase in the efficiency of the function of the kidneys. All of this begins with the voluntary increase of the efficiency of the function of the diaphragm.

Heart and Kidney Communication

It appears that the heart communicates with the kidneys, and they work as a team in the moving and filtering of blood. When we voluntary contract our diaphragm beyond the involuntary contraction, we then increase the volume of blood that returns to the heart. This increased volume of blood that is returned to the heart will fortunately be the volume of blood that will be ejected from the heart.

Once the heart receives this increased volume of blood, it will cause a stretching of the heart muscle cells. The heart will then alert the kidneys that there is an increase in the volume of blood to be received, so then the kidneys prepare themselves to increase their capacity of filtering this increased volume of blood.

Increasing the Efficiency of the Diaphragm

Keep in mind when you increase the efficiency of the function of the diaphragm, it leads to the increase in the efficiency of the lungs. When you increase the efficiency of the lungs, it leads to the increase in the efficiency of the heart. When you increase the efficiency of the heart, it leads to the increase in the efficiency of the kidneys.

Stated another way, if you maximize the function of the diaphragm, then you maximize the function of the lungs. When you maximize the function of the lungs, then you maximize the function of the heart. When you maximize the function of the heart, then you maximize the function of the kidneys.

Further maximizing of the heart function leads to activating parasympathetic nerve activity. It is important to understand that the increase in the efficiency of the lungs, heart, and kidneys are all "involuntary functions" but heavily influenced by the "voluntary" function of the diaphragm.

In addition, the hormone atrial natriuretic peptide (ANP) not only makes your kidneys function more efficiently, but it also modifies the function of the kidneys to function as a natural diuretic. Correlating that when the heart functions more efficiently, it directly stimulates the kidneys' function to become more efficient. When the the kidneys' function become more efficient, the function of the kidneys resembles the function in response to a diuretic.

The Diaphragm's Function as a Natural Diuretic

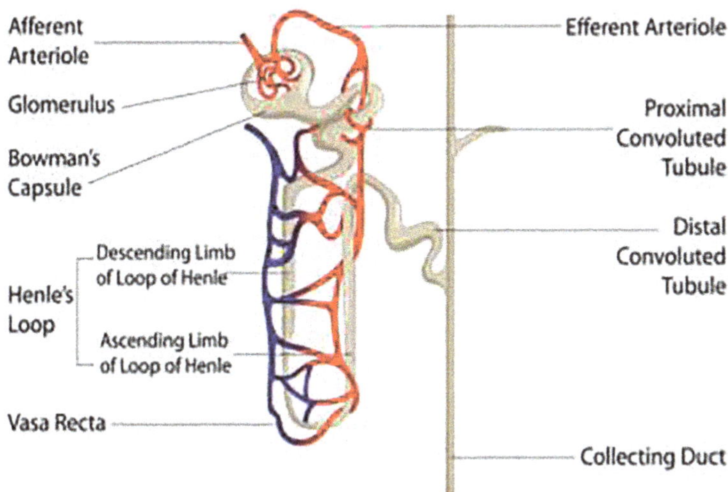

I will now discuss how the diaphragm can act as a natural diuretic for your kidneys. *The focus on this section will be on the renal tubule.* Diuretic activity is known to rid the body of water and salt.

Introduction

When the contraction of the diaphragm is maximized or contracted beyond the involuntary contraction of the diaphragm, which is the contraction of the diaphragm that occurs during normal or "quiet breathing," it generates a greater compression against the inferior vena cava. The inferior vena cava is a large vein that is very close to and runs directly into right atrium of the heart. The vena cava also receives blood from all the other veins of the middle and lower parts of the body before the venous blood returns to the heart. This maximization of the contraction of the diaphragm also generates a greater compression against the thoracic duct. The thoracic duct is the largest lymphatic vessel in the human body. Lymphatic vessels contain lymph. Lymph consists of filtered water and dissolved filtrates that must be returned to the blood, as well as consist of circulating cells of the immune system.

This greater compression by the diaphragm against the vena cava causes an increase in the volume of blood that returns to the heart via the right atrium. This greater compression by the diaphragm against the thoracic duct also causes an increase in the volume of lymphatic fluid that returns to the heart via the right atrium. This increased volume of blood and fluid that returns to the heart leads to an increase in the stretching of the heart (cardiac) muscle cells of the right atrium. This increase in the stretching of the heart muscle cells of the right atrium will stimulate the secretion of the hormone called **atrial natriuretic peptide (ANP)**. It is this hormone, atrial natriuretic peptide, that once released from the heart cells will travel to the kidneys, act on the kidneys, and create the conditions for the kidneys to expel more salt and water in the urine, hence, the effects of a diuretic.

When atrial natriuretic peptide (ANP) is "deployed" and acts on the kidneys, quite a few things happen. The first thing that happens is the glomerular filtration rate (GFR) or basically the kidney filtration rate increases. This increase occurs by way of increasing the surface area of the kidney's filtration membrane (glomerular capillaries). The kidney's filtration membrane is maximized as a result of the relaxation of the mesangial cells in their response to the presence of ANP. This increase of the surface area of the kidneys' glomerular capillary filtration membrane allows for an increase in the volume of available filtrate/fluid. This filtrate/fluid has the potential to become urine. It contains water, ions, salt, wastes, toxins, etc., to be available for reabsorption or excretion. This increase in the volume of available filtrate/fluid then sets the stage for the possible excretion of a larger volume of water and a larger amount of salt than usual, creating the possibility of a greater urine output.

Once this larger volume of filtrate is generated by the renal corpuscle, it then passes through a structure called the renal tubule. The renal tubule consists of a series of structures that determine what substances in the kidney filtrate will be reabsorbed, excreted, or if anything else, be secreted for excretion as well. The structures in the renal tubule that the kidney filtrate passes through before becoming urine include the following in this respective order: **(1)** a proximal convoluted tubule, **(2)** a loop of Henle (nephron loop), **(3)** a distal convoluted tubule, and **(4)** a collecting duct, where many distal convoluted tubules contribute into.

1.) The Proximal Convoluted Tubule

The proximal convoluted tubule is the first structure that the kidney filtrate passes through. The proximal convoluted tubule is responsible for reabsorption of water and many of the filtered solutes back to the bloodstream and makes the largest contribution to reabsorption of the kidney's filtrate.

In general, the proximal convoluted tubule reabsorbs about 65 percent of the filtered water (H_2O), sodium (natrium, Na), and potassium (kalium, K), 100 percent of most filtered organic solutes such as glucose ($C_6H_{12}O_6$) and amino acids, 50 percent of filtered chloride (Cl), 80 through 90 percent of filtered bicarbonate (HCO_3^-), as well as 50 percent of the filtered urea (CH_4N_2O) and a variable amount of filtered calcium (Ca), magnesium (Mg), and phosphate (PO_4^{3-})

In addition, the proximal convoluted tubule secretes variable amounts of hydrogen ions, ammonium ions and urea. Most solute reabsorption in the proximal convoluted tubule involves sodium.

The proximal convoluted tubule and atrial natriuretic peptide

Atrial natriuretic peptide (ANP) inhibits water and sodium reabsorption in the proximal convoluted tubule. This is the very structure of the renal tubule that normally makes the greatest contribution of the reabsorption of water and salt, which would be 65 percent. This effect, of the inhibition of the reabsorption of water and salt, allows for a larger volume of water and greater amount of salt to be available for excretion in the urine moving forward. This hormone inhibits reabsorption of water and salt only, without interfering with the normal reabsorption of the other necessary solutes. Once the larger volume of filtrate leaves the proximal convoluted tubule, it continues to flow along to the next few structures of the renal tubule that are unaffected by the presence of the atrial natriuretic peptide. Keep in mind that the filtrate still contains most of its water and sodium (salt) at this point.

2.) Loop of Henle

The next structure that the kidney filtrate passes through is called the loop of Henle (nephron loop), which has an initial descending limb followed by an ascending limb. The ascending loop has a thin and thick portion. The function of the loop of Henle remains unchanged by ANP and the descending loop of Henle **reabsorbs about 15 percent of the filtered water,** and the ascending loop of Henle **reabsorbs 20 through 30 percent of the filtered sodium and potassium,** as it is impermeable to water, 35 percent of the filtered chloride, 10 through 20 percent of filtered bicarbonate, and a variable amount of the filtered calcium and magnesium.

3.) Initial Part of the Distal Convoluted Tubule

As the remaining filtrate flows through the thick ascending loop of Henle, the fluid then enters the distal convoluted tubule. The initial part of the distal convoluted tubule (DCT) **reabsorbs about 10 through 15 % of filtered water, 5 percent of the filtered sodium, and** 5 percent of the filtered chloride, unaffected by the presence of atrial natriuretic peptide.

4.) End of Distal Convoluted Tubule and the Collecting Duct (ADH/Aldosterone)

Once the fluid reaches the end of the distal convoluted tubule and collecting duct, the amount of water and solute reabsorption is facultative and varies depending on the body's needs. The ability of the reabsorption of water by the distal convoluted tubule and collecting duct is dependent upon availability/presence of the hormone antidiuretic hormone (ADH) or vasopressin. The ability of reabsorption of sodium in the collecting duct is dependent on the availability of the hormone aldosterone.

End of distal convoluted tubule, the collecting duct, and ANP

Atrial natriuretic peptide (ANP) in addition to inhibiting reabsorption of water and salt at the proximal convoluted tubule also regulates the facultative reabsorption in the end of the distal convoluted tubule and the collecting duct. The presence of antidiuretic hormone enhances the reabsorption of water in the end of the distal convoluted tubule and collecting duct and as a reminder the filtrate or fluid in the collecting duct is a collection from many distal convoluted tubules.

Atrial natriuretic peptide suppresses the secretion of ADH, inhibiting further water reabsorption at the end of the distal convoluted tubule and collecting duct. This maintains a larger volume of water available to be excreted in the urine. The presence of aldosterone enhances the reabsorption of sodium in the collecting duct.

Atrial natriuretic peptide also suppresses the secretion of aldosterone, inhibiting further sodium reabsorption in the collecting duct. This ensures a larger amount of sodium to be available for excretion in the urine as well.

Overall, this increase of water and salt output in the form of urine is the function of a diuretic.

Recap

ANP inhibits water and salt reabsorption at the proximal convoluted tubule. ANP prevents further water and salt (sodium) reabsorption at the end of the distal convoluted tubule and collecting duct by suppressing production of the hormones that are responsible for the facultative reabsorption of water and salt.

Atrial natriuretic peptide suppresses both hormones **ADH** and **aldosterone**, the hormones that together enhance both water and salt reabsorption.

Comparison of the excretion of water and sodium by the kidneys with and without ANP according to the numbers of reabsorption.

Without the presence of ANP, 95 % of water in the kidney filtrate would be reabsorbed leaving 5 % to be excreted. So then if there was **one hundred milliliters** of water in the kidney filtrate, then only **five milliliters would be excreted in the urine.**

Without the presence of ANP, about 90 % to 100 % of the sodium in the kidney filtrate would be reabsorbed, leaving 0 to 10 % of sodium to be excreted. So then if there was one hundred milligrams of sodium in the kidney filtrate, then only **zero to ten milligrams of sodium would be excreted in the urine.**

In the presence of ANP, only about 30 % of the water in the kidney filtrate would be reabsorbed, leaving 70 % to be excreted. So from **one hundred milliliters** of filtered water, **seventy milliliters would be excreted as urine.** 997 In the presence of ANP, only about 25 % to 35 % of the sodium in the kidney filtrate would be reabsorbed, leaving 65 % to 75 % to be excreted. So if there was **one hundred milligrams** of sodium in the kidney filtrate, then about **sixty-five to seventy-five milligrams of sodium would be excreted in the urine.**

The Diaphragm and Aging

Aging has been characterized in one case as "a gradual decline in organ functional reserves, which reduces the ability to maintain homeostasis under conditions of stress." When the body is put under stress, it tries to relieve that stress and the act of relieving that stress requires the input of energy. Another description of aging is that "it is associated with a progressive degeneration of the tissues, which has a negative impact on the structure and function of vital organs and is among the most important known risk factors for most chronic diseases" and "as aging is not a disease itself but increases vulnerability to disease." Another statement addressing aging is "all organs tend to lose function with age and is well described in the lung where there is a progressive decline in lung function after twenty-five years old."

A misconception of this is what lung function is. The lungs provide a medium where gas exchange of oxygen and carbon dioxide occur with the blood. The lungs do nothing else, as it is the diaphragm that has a direct effect on the lungs, so if lung function progressively declines, that may be an indication that the diaphragm function is declining instead. When it comes to aging, the function of the diaphragm's contraction and relaxation cycle or the normal breathing pattern is guided by mostly autonomic, involuntary control. Over time, the breathing becomes more and more shallow. Autonomic (involuntary, unconscious) contraction of the diaphragm or involuntary breathing does not utilize the full potential of contraction of the diaphragm; therefore, it does not maximize the intake of oxygen.

Without the full support of the diaphragm, postural changes may occur, compressing the diaphragm, which may hinder diaphragmatic contraction further. This postural hinderance may go undetected since it may be subtle or gradual. Just like when other skeletal muscles are not strengthened or trained, they get weaker over time, so if the diaphragm is not strengthened, it also gets weaker over time and its function declines as well.

When the function of the diaphragm declines, so does breathing or breath. When the breathing declines, so does the availability of oxygen. When the availability of oxygen declines, so does the amount of available energy generated. When the amount of energy generated in the body declines, the amount of energy to support body function may not be sufficient. If the amount of energy generated is not sufficient, overtime decline in body function may occur. Once this decline in body function is noticeable, it is then viewed as aging.

Function has shown that a somatic (voluntary, conscious) contraction of the diaphragm can maximize the contraction of the diaphragm; therefore, it can maximize oxygen intake. If the contraction of the diaphragm is maximized, then the intake of oxygen will be maximized. If the intake of oxygen is maximized, then the energy produced in the body will be maximized. This maximized amount of energy produced will be provided to sustain efficient function. In consequence, this will make the diaphragm stronger in the process, and in general, your diaphragm should get stronger with age with consistent practice.

It does not take a lot to contract the diaphragm beyond the autonomic/involuntary breathing contraction of the diaphragm. Putting more effort in to the contraction of the diaphragm may reverse or slow some symptoms of the onset of aging, and you have the power to make that happen. People at times talk of searching all around the world for the fountain of youth or rely on supplemental herbs (as herbs are good, too, don't get me wrong) when all that may have to be done is to turn within and access the power of the diaphragm.

The Diaphragm and the Immune System / Oxygen

Introduction

When it comes to illnesses, our bodies are equipped with an immune system, which is our most ready and available form of immunity. Immunity is the ability to ward off damage or disease through our defenses.

There are two forms of immunity, the innate (nonspecific) immunity and adaptive (specific) immunity. Innate immunity refers to the barrier that is designed to prevent microbes from gaining access into the body. The adaptive immunity refers to defenses that involve specific recognition of a microbe once it has breached the innate immunity defenses and has entered the body. The adaptive immunity includes lymphocytes—a type of white blood cell, which include the ones called T lymphocytes (T cells) and B lymphocytes (B cells) that fight off pathogens (bacteria, viruses)—and a system to transport these lymphocytes and other white blood cells.

The Lymphatic System

In this section, I will only focus on adaptive immunity. The system that is responsible for and supports the adaptive immunity is the lymphatic system. The lymphatic system is composed of lymph vessels (and other significant organs such as the spleen) that travel throughout in conjunction with the digestive system and the cardiovascular system. In working with conjunction with the cardiovascular system, the lymphatic system collects filtrate or interstitial fluid from the bloodstream, and this fluid is called lymph. This lymph fluid is created when arterial blood squeezes through the capillaries to become venous blood. The fluid removed from arterial blood that does not return by way of venous blood becomes the filtrate that enters the lymphatic system. The contents of this filtrate or lymph fluid include a small amount of protein, salts, glucose, fats, water, white blood cells, and is very similar to blood plasma. This lymph fluid is filtered as it travels throughout the lymphatic system and is returned to the blood.

The vessels of the lymphatic system connect to lymph nodes in which there are about six hundred of them throughout the body loaded with white blood cells including B cells and T cells known as lymphocytes, macrophages, dendritic cells (DC), and follicular dendritic cells (FDC). The follicular dendritic cells present antigen (viral) components to B cells. Once this antigen component is presented to the B cell, it influences an immune response from the B cell. The dendritic cells present antigen components to T cells. Once this antigen component is presented to the T cell, it influences an immune response from the T cell. The B cells are antibody producing and become memory cells after encountering an antigen. The B cells or antibodies attack antigens that are outside the cells, over long distance. The T cells migrate to areas of the body where there is antigen activity. The T cells then attack the antigens that are located inside infected cells and become memory cells.

In addition to the lymph node functioning as a reservoir of immune cells, it also acts as a filter to trap foreign substances that could pose a possible danger to the human body. If any foreign substance(s) become trapped in the lymph node, some are destroyed by the macrophages by phagocytosis, while others are destroyed by lymphocytes (B and T cells) by immune response.

Support for the Immune System

Unfortunately, the lymphatic system does not have a pump to circulate the lymph fluid, so just like for venous blood return, the lymphatic system depends on skeletal muscle contractions to assist in its circulation of lymph fluid in addition to gravity, even though there is contraction of smooth muscle in the vessel walls. While most of the time major skeletal muscles are not in use, the respiratory pump, the diaphragm, is. I mention this to restore faith in the reliability of natural immunity.

By design, the immune system is a very intelligent, sophisticated, extremely efficient, dependable system capable of destroying many pathogens and is always available, yet it could still use a little more support from the function of the diaphragm. If we become involved in a more sedentary lifestyle, from old age, health complications, or career choice, then the full contraction of the diaphragm becomes even more "essential" for immune function and support, as it is the most reliable skeletal muscle capable of pumping lymph fluid.

If lymph fluid is not properly flowing and too much time passes before the first encounter of an antigen (virus) with the immune system, the discomfort from this perceived delayed reaction may seem as if the immune system is unreliable but that would not be accurate. If we do what we can to keep more lymph fluid flowing and more oxygen available, then the reliability of the immune system should be maintained.

For people that have lots of faith in a vaccine, the method of vaccine function still relies on your immune system to protect you, as the body's response to a vaccine produces an immune response by several methods. It can be from an injection of neutralized virus triggering an immune response or by injection using mRNA to manipulate the cells of the body into producing a viral protein recognized by the immune cells, triggering an immune response.

As vaccines are necessary at times, the vaccine primes the immune system by creating a "primary response" without an actual infection. A primary response is relatively slow, as it is the first encounter with the antigen. The benefit of this is that later, if the actual antigen is detected in the body, it will promote a "secondary response" that is much faster and more aggressive than the "primary response." This immune response is still coming from the function of your immune system. So the function of the vaccine is still dependent upon the response from your immune system. If your immune system was nonfunctioning, then vaccines would not be helpful. For the immune system to still be reliable even with vaccine assistance, it must be taken care of, kept strong, and ready. To do so would require improvement in blood and lymph circulation, as this is key to antigen encounter as well as an increase in oxygen availability to help increase the available energy for function.

We should continue natural practices to strengthen our immune system in conjunction with the support of vaccines. We are designed to be a moving species; however, sometimes we spend most of the time involved in sedentary activities. These activities remove the contractional support of major skeletal muscles. The removal of this contractional support from major skeletal muscles contributes to the decrease in the movement of lymph fluid in conjunction with the decrease in movement of venous blood and decrease in oxygen delivery and waste removal.

Fortunately, in sedentary activities, the movement of lymph fluid can be increased with the function of the diaphragm. The contraction and relaxation of the diaphragm during the breathing cycle contributes to the movement of lymph fluid, and the degree of contraction determines how much lymph fluid gets circulated.

The Voluntary Contraction of the Diaphragm and Immunity

The full or maximum voluntary contraction of the diaphragm generates a movement of a greater volume of lymph fluid through the lymphatic system than a normal regular involuntary contraction of the diaphragm. It will also generate a movement of a greater volume of blood as well. Not only does the greater contraction of the diaphragm generate a greater movement of lymph fluid and blood, but it also brings in a greater amount of oxygen.

This increase in the amount of movement of lymph fluid will allow lymph nodes to be more efficient at trapping foreign particles. This increase in the amount of movement of lymph fluid will allow the presence of white blood cells in the lymph nodes to be more efficient at increasing the rate of contact with foreign (viral) particles, leading to a more immediate immune response. The increase in the amount of movement of lymph fluid as a transportation system for the white blood cells will allow the immune cells to be more efficient at patrolling the body, deploying antibodies, and deploying cells looking to attack other cells containing viral material. The increase in blood and oxygen delivery will increase the energy production for all immune cells, as select ones will become more efficient at proliferation (making more copies) and antibody production.

Ensuring the availability of sufficient energy to support the function of immune cell activity can ensure sufficient protection. Upon relaxation of the diaphragm, a greater amount of metabolic wastes would be removed in exhalation. An increase in waste removal is beneficial for immunity by removing substances that could potentially interfere with energy production in the body.

Summary

As more fluid is pumped through the lymphatic system at a greater rate, more lymph fluid is filtered at a greater rate as it flows through the lymph nodes. When more fluid is filtered at a greater rate through the lymph nodes, it increases the rate of contact between antigens (viruses) with white blood cells, decreasing the time between antigen entry of the body and first contact with the immune system. This contributes to the potential of a more immediate immune response, leading to the elimination and filtering of pathogens while minimizing or preventing a symptomatic illness.

The longer an antigen remains in the body undetected, the greater the potential for complications created from its viral activities. So it is beneficial to pump as much fluid as possible throughout the lymphatic system, and the diaphragm can increase the rate at which lymph fluid flows through the lymphatic system, but it must be voluntarily engaged.

The Diaphragm Assists the Spleen

The full or maximum contraction of the diaphragm increases the movement of blood. This increase in the flow of blood will increase the flow of blood entering the spleen, which is part of the lymphatic system. The spleen acts like a lymph node, but for the blood instead of lymphatic fluid..

Sometimes illness is viewed as some level of deficiency of oxygen on the cellular level. If this is the case at times, then there may be a simple inexpensive remedy from the voluntary full contraction of the diaphragm. In addition, "oxygen" is naturally selective in what it kills. Unlike drugs and antibiotics, it does not harm the anaerobic, or beneficial bacteria, which are essential for good health. Only oxygen can selectively kill the bad bacteria without killing the good.

The Diaphragm and Life

I would like to mention again how important it is for us to take in oxygen to support life. Oxygen consumption powers just about all the functions in our bodies to sustain life. The greatest gift to life is oxygen because without it, life for us would not exist. Some say there is nothing greater than the gift of life, and the greatest gift to life is oxygen. If we really cherish life, then the greatest gift we can give ourselves is limitless access to oxygen, as it is what powers life. The more oxygen we give ourselves, then the more life and spirit we give ourselves. The more life that we give ourselves with our intake of oxygen, the more life will give back to us experienced in our quality of life. That should motivate us to strive for cleaner air, cleaner water, and healthier food. As it is very healthy to take a full breath, it should be coordinated along with drinking clean water and eating clean/healthy foods.

In saying that, if we want the maximum benefits that life can give us, then we should never limit ourselves to our availability of oxygen or place physical limitations on our flow of oxygen and allow the power of life to combat death, even when death comes in the form of a virus. Life is stronger than death, and we are put here to live. We are designed to resist death, but we need to access more oxygen through the power of the diaphragm. Maximizing oxygen intake requires that our air passages be clear, giving the body a fair chance to try and protect itself, preserving us as a species in the process. And it will.

Your body will never give up on you if you continue to support it, and the way you support it is by not placing limitations on its oxygen availability. Placing limitations on our oxygen availability is done either by constricting air passageways and/or not engaging the diaphragm to its full potential. We cannot maximize our lives while limiting our oxygen intake while we wear physical restraints over our mouth and nose, which occurs while wearing masks. So every possible chance we are able to take in a maximum breath unrestricted should be a priority. I personally think the diaphragm and the breath is stronger than any virus but always stay safe and err on the side of caution..

The Diaphragm and Entropy (Chaos)

In chemistry, I learned that spontaneous chemical reactions generally have a natural tendency to favor reactions that increase in entropy. And entropy is a measure of chaos, disorder, or randomness. I will use the term chaos moving forward. Since these reactions generally happen spontaneously, they do not require much energy input. However, for chemical reactions to counteract the effects of chaos and restore order, an input of energy is needed. These kinds of chemical reactions also occur in the human body. Life in this case can be viewed as a balance between reactions that cause order and chaos. The young if measured by the concept of chaos can be considered as having a greater rate for chemical reactions maintaining order than the rate of the chemical reactions generating chaos. Aging or getting old if measured by the concept of chaos would indicate that the chemical reactions creating chaos are occurring at a greater rate than the chemical reactions generating order. The reactions that counter chaos and restore order require inputs of energy. In order to introduce more input of energy, more oxygen would have to be made available for the body, and in order to do this, more breath must be taken into the body. This can only occur by more engagement of the diaphragm, which would come from conscious voluntary breathing. Therefore, this may indicate that conscious voluntary breathing may be a good weapon to resist this natural tendency toward chaos.

Our lives are believed to end once our bodies achieve total chaos. The manifestation of total chaos would mean our total input of energy was not efficient enough to resist the changes created by chaos. The purpose of breathing is to preserve life, so therefore, breathing must be the way to resist chaos. As breathing gets shallow, then the level or quality of life decreases and the level of chaos increases, and as the breathing gets deeper and stronger, then the quality of life increases and the level of chaos decreases. And this level of breathing is available through the power of the diaphragm when voluntarily engaged.

In a world of chaos, you may notice that the focus is not on encouraging people to increase their health and performance by way of increasing oxygen consumption nor is the focus on the diaphragm. Other artificial measures are encouraged to be used instead to combat chaos. This could mean that even in a society and not just the body that not maximizing the input of oxygen first can lead to chaos. When someone is in panic mode, the person is instructed to relax and breathe. Even in that situation, it shows that when oxygen levels in the brain is poor, it creates chaos in the brain and rather quickly.

The Diaphragm and Massage Therapy

First, I would like to say that massage therapy is more of a medical necessity than it is a luxury. For reasons that people go to the doctor for concern of health, people should frequent massage therapy for some of the same reasons. As long as the methods used in massage therapy increase the rate of blood flow and lymph fluid flow, then you are receiving health benefits.

The practice of massage therapy in most cases use manual manipulation of the body's soft tissues to not only release muscle tension, stress, and pain but to also move blood and lymph throughout the body. The effect from the increase in the movement of blood and lymphatic fluid will give you similar benefits as to what the diaphragm's full contraction provides, greater venous blood return to the heart, and support for immune function by the increased circulation of lymph fluids. With increased blood return to the heart, increased lymph flow, as well as increased muscle relaxation, health increases and medical complications decrease in addition to parasympathetic nerve activity engagement.

Another good thing about massage therapy is that you get the same benefits as full diaphragmatic contraction from the efforts of someone else and the diaphragm can relax a little more during that time!

The Diaphragm and the Feet

I would like to talk about a personal experience I have had with my feet and the diaphragm. As long as I could remember, I have always had issues with my toes feeling numb when they were massaged. My feet felt fine otherwise. I was aware that the feeling of numbness had to do with a circulation issue. But I did not know why I had a circulation issue.

During the year 2019, I began to have problems with my feet and had difficulty standing on them for very long. I would say that after about an hour or two, tops, my feet began to really hurt and feel irritated. At the time, I was working as a massage therapist, and it became very frustrating. It began to become difficult to perform the trade after one or two clients, and I was hoping to perform five to seven treatments in a day. After one or two treatments, my feet would feel like they were on fire. I began to assume that I had plantar fasciitis yet not diagnosed.

I began to apply and practice my theory of the voluntary maximum contraction of the diaphragm. I attempted to use the effects of maximizing oxygen input along with maximizing blood and fluid circulation to see whether it would be beneficial for my feet. I know that the maximum contraction of the diaphragm maximizes blood flow and oxygen input.

Every day following, in the morning, I would hydrate then stand and maximize the contraction of the diaphragm and let the relaxation of the diaphragm guide itself repetitiously for thirty minutes to an hour minimum. My rationale in choosing to stand was because I wanted to use gravity to pull the blood down to my feet with less kinks in the blood vessels as you may find in sitting and then use the power of the diaphragm to pull the blood out of my feet and legs by drawing the blood up into the heart upon the full or maximum contraction of the diaphragm repeatedly.

Week by week, I would get better at it. After about a month, I no longer had the irritation sensation in the feet and any discomfort I would feel felt like normal aches, but I would not feel discomfort in my feet until after standing on them for about four or five hours. I still practice diaphragm strengthening until this day. Also, during my most recent massage in 2021, it surprised me when my toes no longer felt numb when massaged. They felt normal.

My standing stance: I had feet shoulder-width apart, knees slightly bent, slight pelvic tuck, elongated thoracic spine, slight lift in the collar bones, elongated cervical spine, chin tucked down, and ears drawn back in line with the shoulders.

I would also like to add.

There was an article published on June 30, 2021 (date) at University of Colorado Boulder (source).

Summary: A new study shows that a breathing exercise known as inspiratory muscle strength training (IMST) can reduce blood pressure in weeks, with benefits on par with daily exercise or medication.

Other statements from the article: Five-minute breathing workout lowers blood pressure as much as exercise and drugs and "strength training for breathing muscles" holds promise for host of health benefits ("5-minute Workout Lowers Blood Pressure as Much as Exercise, Drugs," https://www.colorado.edu). This article was written by Lisa Marshall.

Experiences that Contributed to My Realization of the Diaphragm's Importance

1. I was told by a former classmate that holding the qi gong postures made me very powerful.
2. Someone said many years ago that I said that the most important muscle to exercise is your diaphragm.
3. The last thing my late kung fu teacher told me to do before he passed away was "do three hundred breaths a day kid."
4. I observed and recognized that the diaphragm rarely gets fatigued, and during strenuous runs, it works hard and never quits.
5. I noticed that when I returned to static training that my diaphragm was the only muscle that was trying to work harder for me to hold the postures as my other muscles began to feel fatigued and give out. The diaphragm did not.
6. We continuously breathe and can only stop ourselves from breathing for so long.
7. My kung fu teacher told me that I was not breathing right when I began to feel fatigued.

Energy Cycle for Glucose, Fatty Acids, and Ketone Bodies (All require oxygen for complete oxidation.)

(All require oxygen for complete oxidation.)

The need for oxygen is for the continuous production of energy in the form of ATP (energy) from glucose

(**A.** glycolysis, **B.** Krebs cycle, **C.** electron transport chain [ETC]) summarized here in three steps **(A, B, C)**:

(A) glycolysis: glucose breakdown for energy (no oxygen needed)

Step one: glucose ($C_6H_{12}O_6$)→ Pyruvate ($C_3H_4O_3$) + ATP + NADH + H+

Step two A (no oxygen [O2] available): Pyruvate + NADH → lactic acid / lactate ($C_3H_6O_3$) + H+ + NAD+ (burning sensation)

Step two B (oxygen is available): Pyruvate → acetyl-CoA + CO_2

(B) Krebs cycle (only when oxygen [O^2]) is readily available): acetyl-CoA →NADH + H+ + $FADH_2$ + GTP + CO_2

(C) electron transport chain (ETC) (O_2 available): NADH + H+ + $FADH_2$ + O_2 → ATP (lots of it) + H_2O

Long-chain fatty acids cannot cross the blood-brain barrier, but the liver can beak these down to produce ketone bodies (acetone, acetoacetic acid, beta-hydroxybutyric acid). However, short-chained fatty acids (e.g., butyric acid, propionic acid, and acetic acid) and the medium-chained fatty acids (octanoic acid, heptanoic acid, and hexanoic acid) can cross the blood-brain barrier and be metabolized by brain cells.

Fatty-Acid (Beta Oxidation) Metabolism

Step one: fatty-acid ($CH_3(CH_2)COOH$) → acetyl-CoA

Step two: acetyl-CoA → NADH + $FADH_2$ + GTP + CO_2 – Krebs Cycle

Step three: NADH + $FADH_2$ + O_2 → ATP (lots of it) + H_2O – ETC

Ketone Body Metabolism

Step one: ketone Body ($C_4H_4O_3$) → acetyl-CoA

Step two: acetyl-CoA → NADH + $FADH_2$ + GTP + CO_2 – Krebs Cycle

Step three: NADH+ $FADH_2$ + O_2 → ATP (lots of it) + H_2O – ETC

Another look at lactic acid (Oxygen available):

Step two A (in reverse): lactic Acid/lactate + NAD+ → Pyruvate + NADH

Summary of Oxygen Requiring Chemical Reactions

Glucose gets metabolized to pyruvate without the need of oxygen. If no oxygen is available, then pyruvate gets reversibly converted to lactic acid. When oxygen is available, pyruvate is converted to acetyl-CoA and goes through a series of reactions that require oxygen, producing maximum amounts of energy in the form of molecules of ATP. Fatty acids are broken down to molecules of acetyl-CoA upon metabolism, also going through a series of reactions that require oxygen to maximize ATP output. Ketone bodies are converted to acetyl-CoA upon metabolism, going through the same process that is previously detailed. These reactions require oxygen for complete metabolism for the final output of large amounts of energy (ATP).

Muscular Contraction in Necessity of ATP

With available ATP, the contraction cycle of the muscle cell involves four steps:

1. ***ATP hydrolysis.*** ATP is hydrolyzed to ADP, energizing the myosin head (ATP → ADP + P + energy)
2. ***Attachment of myosin to actin to form cross bridges.*** The energized myosin head attaches to the myosin-binding site on actin, releasing the previously hydrolyzed phosphate group (-P).
3. ***Power stroke.*** The crossbridge then rotates releasing ADP, generating force as it rotates toward the center of the sarcomere.
4. ***Detachment of myosin from actin.*** At the end of the power stroke, the cross bridge remains firmly attached to actin until it binds a molecule of ATP. Upon binding a new molecule of ATP, the myosin head detaches and the muscle can relax again.

The diaphragm. A dome-shaped muscle that separates the thoracic cavity from the abdominopelvic cavity. The diaphragm is the most important muscle that powers breathing. The diaphragm has a convex superior surface that forms the floor of the thoracic cavity and a concave, inferior surface that forms the roof of the abdominal cavity. The peripheral muscular portion of the diaphragm originates on the xiphoid process of the sternum, the inferior six ribs and their costal cartilages, and the lumbar vertebrae and their intervertebral discs and the twelfth rib. From their various origins, the fibers of the muscular portion converge and insert into the central tendon, a strong aponeurosis located near the center of the muscle. The central tendon fuses with the inferior surface of the pericardium (covering of the heart) and the pleurae (coverings of the lungs). The two halves of the diaphragm can work on its own if necessary due to a paralysis—unpaired skeletal muscle.

Muscles of inhalation include the diaphragm and the external intercostals.

Muscles of exhalation include the diaphragm.

Muscles of forced inhalation include the diaphragm, external intercostals, sternocleidomastoid, scalenes, and the pec minor.

Muscles of forced exhalation include the diaphragm, the external oblique, internal oblique, transverse abdominis, rectus abdominis, and internal intercostals.

The nonrespiratory functions of the diaphragm include help in vomiting and throwing up and expulsion of feces and urine from the body. It also prevents acid reflux by exertion of pressure on the esophagus when it passes through the esophageal hiatus.

Sources

Dreha-Kulaczewski, Steffi; Joseph, Arun A.; Merboldt, Klaus-Dietmar; Ludwig, Hans-Christoph; Gartner, Jutta; and Frahm, Jens. "Inspiration is the major regulator of human CSF flow." J Neurosci 35(6) (February 2015):2485-91.

Maciocia, Giovanni, and Xin Ming, Su. The Foundations of Chinese Medicine: A Comprehensive Text for Acupuncturists and Herbalists. New York: Elsevier Churchill Livingstone, 2005. Tortora, Gerard, and Derrickson, Bryan. Principles of Anatomy and Physiology. New Jersey: John Wiley & Sons, Inc.,2009 University of Colorado at Boulder. "5-minute breathing workout lowers blood pressure as much as exercise, drugs: 'Strength training for breathing muscles' holds promise for host of health benefits."

ScienceDaily. ScienceDaily, 30 June 2021. www.sciencedaily.com/releases/2021/06/210630135033.htm.

www.ingramcontent.com/pod-product-compliance
Lightning Source LLC
Chambersburg PA
CBHW052119030426
42335CB00025B/3053
9781961254633